Reversing Memory Loss

Also by the authors

Brain Power

Reversing Memory Loss

Proven Methods for Regaining, Strengthening, and Preserving Your Memory

Fully revised and updated

Vernon H. Mark, M.D.
with Jeffrey P. Mark, M.Sc.

Houghton Mifflin Company   *Boston   New York*

For Alexandra

For Dad

For information about permission to reproduce selections from
this book, write to Permissions, Houghton Mifflin Company,
215 Park Avenue South, New York, New York 10003.

Library of Congress Cataloging-in-Publication Data
Mark Vernon H., date.
   Reversing memory loss: proven methods for regaining, strengthening,
and preserving your memory / Vernon H. Mark, with Jeffrey P. Mark. —
Fully rev. and updated.
      p.   cm
   includes bibliographical references and index.
   ISBN 0-395-94452-x
   1. Memory disorders — Prevention. 2. Memory disorders in old age —
Prevention. 3. Memory. I. Mark, J. Paul. II. Title.
RC394.M46 M37 2000
616.8'4 — dc21   99-046574

Printed in the United States of America

QUM 10 9 8 7 6 5 4

The information presented in case histories and stories in *Reversing Memory Loss*
is medically accurate. However, all names, places, and characteristics that could
identify specific individuals have been changed to protect privacy. Some case histories contain elements from more than one patient. Any resemblance to persons
living or dead is coincidental.

Before you start the regimens presented in this book, consult your own physician to make sure that they are suitable for you.

None of the information presented here is intended to substitute for medical
advice. If you have any problems or questions related to your own health and
fitness, you should direct them to your physician.

Acknowledgments

WITH THE FIRST EDITION of this book, we were fortunate to have had Ruth K. Hapgood as our editor. We are keenly aware that few authors ever have the help of such a gifted editor, or one who brings as much knowledge, enthusiasm, and dedication to her work as Ruth. It has been our pleasure and privilege to revisit the book in this second edition with her, and we thank her for making the manuscript vastly better and more interesting.

We are also grateful to numerous talented individuals at Houghton Mifflin, including Liz Duvall, manuscript editing supervisor, and Christine Graunas, copy editor. And we wish to give special thanks to Rux Martin, senior editor, who shepherded us through the process of revising the first edition and without whose help this new edition would not have been possible.

We are extremely happy to have Flip Brophy of Sterling Lord Literistic represent us, and we thank her for her timely advice and assistance.

I am pleased to have the chance to thank my friend, partner, and colleague, Dr. Thomas D. Sabin. Although neither of us will admit to being that old, our collaboration has now spanned more than thirty years. I feel very fortunate to have worked with Tom, one of the top neurologists in the world, for so long.

As always, I am grateful for the talents of Joyce Sabin of Sabin

Acknowledgments

& Mark, who has guided our enterprise through difficult times. I'd also like to thank Elec Toth and Mary Grace Neal, who have helped Sabin & Mark (both the company and the doctors themselves) in so many ways.

Dr. Jonathan Lieff has been a good friend and trusted associate for a number of years, and I am proud that he has written the foreword to this book.

All errors in fact or judgment are exclusively my own.

Vernon H. Mark, M.D.

Contents

Contents

Foreword

In my experience as a geriatric psychiatrist, memory loss is the reason most people in nursing homes are unable to live independently. Whether that loss is the result of depression, metabolic disturbance, malnutrition, Alzheimer's disease, multi-infarct dementia, stroke, tumor, or any of a variety of major brain injuries or diseases, the result is the same. Without the ability to remember, without the storehouse of memories that allow us to carry out routine functions of daily living, we lose our independence.

America is undeniably getting older. Within the next twenty years many in the "baby boom" generation of the late 1940s and early 1950s will be at the age where they may need to enter nursing homes. But America's nursing homes are already overcrowded, and many are unable to provide the complex of treatment needed for the many different types of patients. Is the solution to build more nursing homes? The answer is really a new vision of care for the elderly and new ways of keeping elderly people out of nursing homes as long as possible. This is the promise of the broader view expressed in *Reversing Memory Loss*.

My initial exposure to Dr. Mark's work came more than twelve years ago when he consulted with several patients that I was treating in nursing homes. Since then I have observed his comprehensive evaluations of many patients. Dr. Mark has had extensive experience in treating the elderly and has studied the issues of nursing home care in great detail. At his Center for Memory Impairment and Neurobehavioral Disorders (CMIND), he coordinated the work of a multidisciplinary team of professionals providing the types of treatment described in this book.

Dr. Mark has always impressed me with his great depth of knowledge about medicine and about his patients. He has the qualities that I respect most in a physician, that is, the ability to concentrate on, and creatively study, all of a patient's relevant symptoms; the vision to pay special attention to the way these many details impinge upon a patient's life; and the energy to care enough about his patients to help them change. In evaluating the brain, and especially the complex disorders of memory, this type of concern is vital.

We are truly at a crossroads in medicine and history. The explosion of information, a result of billions of dollars spent on research, will soon pay enormous dividends. Soon various forms of heart disease and cancer may be entirely curable. As important as those problems are, we must never lose sight of the fact that the brain is ultimately what controls life, and it is our ability to remember that permits us to thrive. *Reversing Memory Loss* prods us to keep medical progress in perspective. What use is a perfectly healthy heart if the brain is unable to remember how to cross a street without being hit by a car?

Alexander Smith once wrote, "A man's real possession is his memory. In nothing else is he rich, in nothing else is he poor." *Reversing Memory Loss* will help everyone who reads it to protect their most vital possession. It contains the collected wisdom of hundreds of medical experts and the most up-to-the-minute information on what each of us can do to reverse the processes that cause memory loss.

I encourage everyone, young and old, to take this book to heart and to make the changes that can lead to a healthier, happier, and more productive life.

JONATHAN D. LIEFF, M.D.

President, American Association for Geriatric Psychiatry (1990–1991)

Fellow, American Psychiatric Association

Associate Clinical Professor of Psychiatry, Boston University Medical School

Diplomate of the American Board of Psychiatry and Neurology, with Added Qualification in Geriatric Psychiatry

Chief of Psychiatry, Arbor Senior Care

INTRODUCTION

Take Charge of Your Life

ARE YOU HAVING TROUBLE remembering things? Do the names of people you've met a dozen times suddenly escape you? Do you ever come into a room to perform a specific task and forget what you wanted to do? You're not alone. Many millions of people share your complaints, and hundreds of thousands regularly worry that they're losing their memories (the first sign, they think, that they're losing their minds), to the point that they seek professional medical advice.

Let me reassure you that the overwhelming majority of these complaints are not associated with Alzheimer's disease or irreversible memory loss. Even if you feel that your memory loss persists, you should not become fearful that the meaningful period of your life has suddenly ended. What you may need to do is undergo medical testing to find out what's wrong, then have the underlying problem corrected. The important thing for you to keep in mind is that many kinds of memory loss can be easily diagnosed and treated.

As you'll learn, there are many different kinds of memory, all of which are controlled by the brain, and all of which are important. However, one kind of memory is essential. It is at the center or core of memory; indeed, it is at the core of your being, representing the essential you, your personality, your

1

feelings. It is called vital memory, and all other forms of memory are rooted in this function.

Sometimes it's difficult to understand how crucial vital memory is in our lives until we see what happens when it's destroyed. In early 1990, a woman testified before Congress about a weight-loss program her forty-five-year-old husband had enrolled in less than a year before. He had been about thirty pounds overweight, and the weight-loss clinic put him on a liquid diet that did, in fact, cause him to shed his unwanted pounds. But one day when the man was out jogging he suddenly had a stroke, the result of the kind of diet he was on, which left him in a coma. Even though he was at first paralyzed and unable to speak, intensive therapy over a period of several months improved his speech and arm and leg functions to the point that he was almost normal. He was left, however, with one critical deficiency: he had lost his vital memory. He had lost all memory of prior events, including who he was, who his wife and children were, and what had been his hopes and dreams for the future.

The man's wife was justifiably bitter. Without his vital memory, she explained, he looked the same, spoke in the same way, and did many things as he had before. Yet he was only a shadow of his former self — a Hollywood facade with no underlying structure. When his vital memory had gone, all the things that made him a unique individual also disappeared. His body was rehabilitated; his mind was not.

Such selective loss of vital memory following a stroke is very uncommon. What this man's experience illustrates, however, is not just that a stroke can be tremendously debilitating, but that his stroke could have been prevented with proper precautions. Moreover, other kinds of memory loss, even those associated with some strokes, can be reversed.

This book is about memory, but it is unlike others that address the topic. Books such as *Thirty Days to a Better Memory*, *Business Success Through Memory*, and *New Secrets of Improving*

Your Memory — and literally hundreds of others of the same variety — are clearly helpful to those of us who want to improve intellectual capacity. But such improvements, nice as they are, are trivial compared to preserving vital memory and reversing the loss of our selves.

Vital memory is one of the most basic and necessary functions of our brains. The cartoonist Gary Larson captured the essence of vital memory in one of his "Far Side" cartoons. An elderly man with a stubble of whiskers wakes up in the morning. Beside the man's bed is a large poster with block letters reminding him, PUT YOUR PANTS ON BEFORE THE SHOES! When you wake up each morning, do you know where you are, who you are, and what the date is? Do you remember what happened the day before, and how it affected you? Do you have a general idea of how you fit into your surroundings? Most important, do you know what your plans and expectations for the immediate future are — the rest of the morning, the afternoon, the evening, tomorrow?

If you retain your vital memory, you will continue to be in charge of your own life. If you don't, life will not have much meaning for you. You become an object rather than a person, someone to be taken care of. The less vital memory you have, the more your individual freedom is compromised. As long as you retain your vital memory you are a going concern, no matter how old you are. Even if some of your memory resources are reduced, or if your visual or hearing memories are diminished, you'll still be able to take care of yourself.

The reason I stress vital memory as the core of your memory function is to give you some perspective on your memory complaints. The more superficial aspects of memory may be deficient from time to time in all of us — you and me included. And when you have problems such as difficulty in recalling a name, forgetting the context of a conversation, having an idea pop into your head and leave just as quickly, you should not be unduly alarmed as long as your vital memory is intact.

Introduction

This book touches on a number of aspects of memory and memory loss, but the subject of vital memory is a recurring theme because it is relevant to every facet of memory. In instances of memory loss, we'll go into the diagnostic steps necessary to find the root cause of the memory problem. More often than not, a helpful treatment is available that is capable of reversing the memory loss and many of the symptoms that go with it.

Keep in mind, however, that human memory is highly subjective and fragile. As you age, you may begin to have some difficulty in remembering, for example, names, particularly when your catalogue or library of memories is very extensive. But if your brain is free from disease or injury, your vital memory should remain intact even into advanced old age.

To make certain that you understand the memory process, I want to discuss in a general way the components of memory so that you can tell the difference between the more and less essential aspects of remembering. I'll also try to give you some information that will help you enhance your ability to remember, even if something has already happened to you to decrease your memory.

I've been fortunate to participate in a revolution in medical science which has brought about major breakthroughs in treating people for loss of vital memory. Thirty years ago I witnessed countless numbers of persons who came to the hospitals where I worked in search of cures for their memory complaints, many of which we were then unable to diagnose, let alone treat. Today a majority of persons with memory problems can be helped. We now know, with certainty, that not all memory loss is permanent, and that there are specific treatments and therapies that can have enormously beneficial results in reversing many kinds of memory loss.

P A R T   I

What Is Vital Memory?

1

How Vital Memory Controls Life

MEMORY IS the most important mental ability we have. It endows us with the facility to learn new things — in fact, it is an essential part of all new learning — and it influences the development of individual behavior. I'm sure you are aware of the fact that some of us have naturally superior language skills, or mathematical ability, or musical and artistic talents. Even athletic skills are dependent on certain kinds of brain development. But without the capacity to remember, none of those innate skills and talents would be of any use.

Superimposed on genetic endowment, which expresses itself in the structure of the brain and its functional and electrochemical powers, is the fact that the brain changes in response to experiences. This ability of the brain to change with experience is called plasticity. And the fact that the brain does change, allowing our behavior to be modified by cues in our surroundings, is a function of memory. The memories laid down by experience influence current and future behavior.

By these environmental cues I mean not only visual and auditory signals — that is, the signals received by the brain through sight and sound — but also the influences of touch, smell, and taste. When these cues are received in the brain, even though they may be largely in one of the five forms of sensation, mixing or integration always occurs, resulting in a composite record of the whole experience. This record is stored chemically in brain tissue. It becomes a physical part of the brain, and is in fact what we call a memory.

The storage site in the brain varies depending on the predominant sensation of the memory. When you remember a beautiful painting you saw in someone's house, that visual memory is related to the visual cortex of the brain. Likewise, a song you heard on the radio, the sound of a young child's laughter, the noise of an airplane taking off are all auditory memories stored in the auditory cortex. The brain also has specific storage sites for other types of memories.

When I say that memory is the central factor that endows us with the ability to learn, I'm talking about the images and impressions of experiences which are sent to the brain by various sense organs, including the senses of vision and hearing, and which give our surroundings life and meaning. The brain's structure is genetically determined, but even on a microscopic level there is evidence that plasticity as a response to environmental stimuli influences the organization of the brain. As a result of this influence, individual behavior, emotional response, and personality develop in a unique way. That's what differentiates one person from another.

Vital memory is the core or center of the memory process, and it is usually the most protected part of memory. Other more superficial types of memory can decrease before vital memory begins to fail. For example, if individuals have had strokes or head injuries, they may have difficulty with vision and even visual memories. But they can nevertheless retain their basic personalities, carry out many functions completely, and lead almost normal lives.

The brain injuries or diseases that alter or destroy some part of vital memory are always severe. Vital memory includes the memories that are laid down earliest in life, such as the knowledge that allows us to live independently and carry out the essential activities of daily living. These memories tell us when it is appropriate to sleep and when to be awake; how and when to get food and drink so that we can sustain our nutritional requirements; where and when to carry out our functions of elimination in a socially acceptable fashion; how to dress ourselves so that we look appropriate in various contexts; how to cross a street without getting hit by a car (quite a complicated undertaking, requiring knowledge of when and where to cross the street as well as some appreciation of the volume and rules of traffic).

Vital memory is necessary in following the rules of safety so that we dispose of smoking materials, avoid fire, and take into account other factors in our surroundings that are likely to be injurious or dangerous. In other words, vital memory is closely tied to basic brain mechanisms necessary for self-preservation. It helps us to know when to fight or run away in the face of danger. And it helps us gauge the appropriateness of our responses in stressful circumstances.

Vital memory contributes to other kinds of behavior. It is important in generating the learned and remembered responses we have to members of our families and the persons we associate with closely every day. It plays an important role in the give-and-take of social conversation and helps us develop the conditioned responses that determine our emotional tone in various situations — for example, our responses to speech or physical contacts from friends or family. Vital memory helps us to adapt and form appropriate social relations, even when we are confronted by strangers.

Finally, vital memory is at the center of all those memories that summarize our life experiences, from our earliest recollections to the present. Taken as a whole, an inventory of these memories lets us know ourselves — who we are and how we fit into our world. Even more important, they define how we became the individuals we are, with our strengths and vulnerabilities, and with our unique personalities and modes of behavior. In other words, the dynamic memories of our past — of who we are — are with us constantly and influence our responses to almost every challenge we face each day, from the time we awaken until we go to sleep. And even then we don't escape them, because they also shape our dreams.

It is easy to confuse some aspects of vital memory with instincts. Most of the behavior that we discuss when we talk about vital memory concerns itself with self-preservation and reproduction. Admittedly, these functions are linked with the basic wiring of the brain. Behavior that avoids pain and seeks pleasure is fundamental to the human condition. Human appetites, such as hunger, thirst, and sexual gratification, are also part of the human repertoire and are associated with the brain. But these basic responses are constantly being modified by experience or, more precisely, by conditioning.

Conditioned responses all relate to a specific memory that is integral to the conditioning process. That doesn't mean that the fight-or-flight response or the arousal of appetite is in itself primarily a memory. The conditioning of these responses, however, always involves memory that modifies and perfects the end product, namely the behavior that we use to preserve our life and our species. The memory that we use to condition our responses to danger or to satisfy our basic appetites is always associated with memories that are tied to strong emotions. In turn, because of the anatomy of the brain, these memories are often associated with unusual smells.

It is not surprising, then, for us to find that the part of the brain associated with vital memory is called the emotional brain or limbic brain. Because of the fact that vital memory is more powerful than any other kind of memory, and in fact controls other memories, it is useful for us to know what the emotional brain is, and why memories associated with it sit in such a commanding position.

Fight-or-flight behavior is one aspect of self-preservation that has existed on this earth for hundreds of millions of years. Indeed, the mechanisms that initiate this kind of behavior are found in the deepest and most primitive centers of the brain. These primitive centers, which are part of our emotional brain, are reflected in the brains of our vertebrate ancestors. Scientists believe that the emotional brain developed about 400 million years ago and flourished 150 million years ago, when reptiles still dominated the earth's crust. Its structures and functions were modified, regulated, and influenced by the "new brain" or "neocortex" that appeared ages later in animals such as the human. The emotional brain is also called the "nose" brain because one of its oldest functions is to detect and interpret odors. Smelling and interpreting odors are hence closely associated in all animals with the emergency responses to a threatening environment.

At first glance, most people assume that the anatomy of the brain is incredibly complicated and all but impossible for the average person to understand. Besides, why would anyone but a doctor or scientist really need to know anything about brain anatomy? The fact is, structure and function are intimately linked, and the more you know about how the brain developed and how it's put together, the better able you'll be to understand the workings of your own brain. I'd therefore like to take you through a brief, but simplified, anatomy lesson, highlighting for you in five diagrams some interesting facts and features.

Throughout this book we will be referring to various parts of the brain, and this section may also help you to better understand where those structures are found and what they're supposed to do. Keep in mind that the brain does not function like a machine. When we look at its anatomy we can't really say that a specific brain structure always and only controls a specific mental function. When we go into more detail about memory, you'll quickly appreciate that numerous parts of the brain control numerous kinds of memory. Don't worry if you don't immediately grasp all the specifics of brain anatomy here. Later on, if you want to go back and locate specific brain structures, the diagrams will serve as handy references.

If we look at a cross section of the brain of an ancient vertebrate, like a crocodile (Figure 1), it shows that practically the
whole brain is the limbic brain. However, again as shown in
Figure 1, a cross section of the human brain discloses it to be

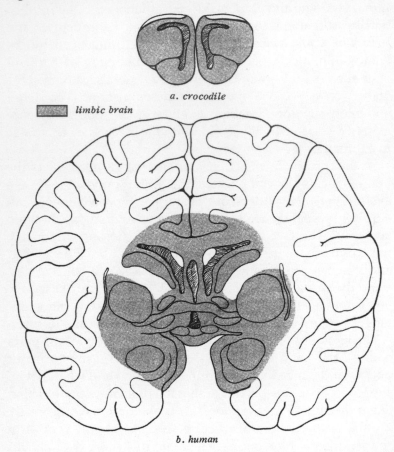

a. crocodile

▨ *limbic brain*

b. human

FIG. 1. A schematic cross section of (*a*) crocodile brain (*b*) human brain.
Coronal (cross) section of human cerebrum is contrasted with section from
crocodile's brain. Limbic portion of both brains darkened by overlay. Crocodile's cerebrum or large brain consists almost entirely of limbic brain, while
markedly greater-sized human brain is accounted for by development of
neocortex or "new brain."

ten times as large as the crocodile brain, and a much smaller part of the brain (shaded area) is the emotional brain. Evolution has pushed the emotional brain close to the brain stem, the tube of neural tissue that connects the large brain to the spinal cord and that controls our vital functions, like respiration, heart rate, and blood pressure.

To give you a better idea about the structure of the brain, Figure 2 shows an outline of the human head and brain in

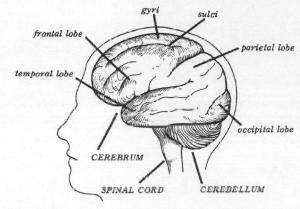

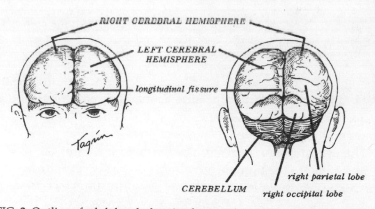

FIG. 2. Outline of adult head, showing brain in lateral, anterior, and posterior views. Surface landmarks of the brain are depicted in side, front, and rear views of the head.

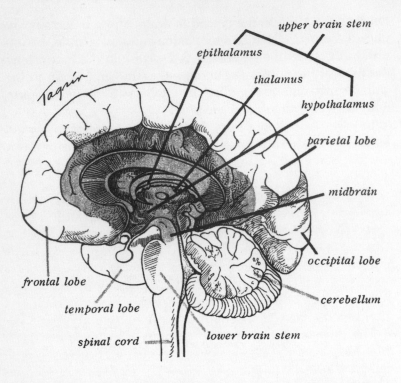

FIG. 3. Medial surface of right cerebral hemisphere and brain stem. Limbic areas of brain are shaded in this sagittal section of *midline* structures which is prepared by separating the two hemispheres and dividing the brain stem lengthwise into two equal parts.

the lateral, anterior, and posterior views. Surface landmarks of the brain are depicted in the side, front, and rear views of the head, including the gyri and sulci, the convolutions on the brain and the spaces between them.

The evolutionary stages of the brain, going from the lower forms of life to the human, are almost precisely reproduced by the human embryo in the womb. The brain starts as a tube of delicate nervous tissue, extending the entire length of the organism. It is protected by the individual bones of the spine and head. That part of the tube that is protected by the backbone evolves into the spinal cord. The part that is protected by the cranium develops into the brain stem.

During the course of evolution, two paired bubbles of brain tissue expanded out of the brain stem on either side. The lower pair formed the *cerebellum*. The upper pair formed the large brain or *cerebrum*. Each half of the cerebrum is itself divided into lobes, named according to their position: the frontal lobe is in the front part of the skull; the occipital lobe is in the back; the parietal lobe is on the top of the brain; and the temporal lobe lies just beneath the temple and ear.

The structures comprising the emotional brain include the upper part of the brain stem as well as the deep structures of the cerebrum. These structures still bear the names given to them by ancient Greek anatomists. Figure 3 shows the midline surface of the right cerebral hemisphere and brain stem. Areas of the emotional brain are shaded in this section of the hemisphere, which is made by separating the two hemispheres and dividing the brain stem lengthwise into two equal parts.

The *thalamus*, which means "an inner bridal chamber," is a place in which the senses (touch, vision, and hearing) can be joined. The epithalamus and hypothalamus are the roof and floor of the thalamus. The limbic brain takes its name from *limbus*, the Latin word for border, since it prominently outlines the inner surface of each cerebral hemisphere. This border is shaped like a letter C. The top of the C is called the *cingulum* (Figure 4), which is the Latin word for girdle or belt. The bottom of the C is called the *hippocampus* because it curls upon itself; if looked at in one way it appears like a sea horse, which is the literal meaning of "hippocampus."

Figure 4 shows a medial surface view of the right cerebral hemisphere with the lower brain stem removed. This gives a clear view of the inner portion of the temporal lobe. Just beneath the *uncus,* near the center of the brain, is an almond-shaped nucleus called the *amygdala,* a structure which helps regulate emotional tone. The *fornix* contains nerve fibers.

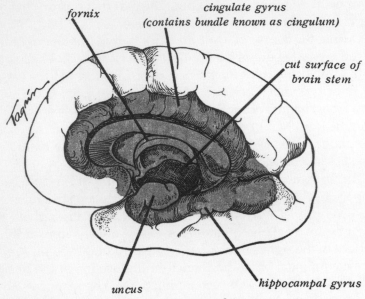

fornix

cingulate gyrus
(contains bundle known as cingulum)

cut surface of
brain stem

hippocampal gyrus

uncus
(thin layer of cortex covering amygdala)

FIG. 4. Medial surface of right cerebral hemisphere (lower brain stem removed). This is another midline view of the brain, but the brain stem has been removed to give a clear view of inner surface of entire cerebral hemisphere, including inner (medial) portion of temporal lobe. Shaded areas are part of limbic system.

Figure 5 shows two cross sections of the brain in two different planes. It shows *ventricles,* fluid-filled spaces inside the brain, and *ganglia,* concentrations of nerve cells. The emotional brain is shaded. These sections allow us to inspect some details of this part of the brain.

The brain is unique among body organs because it does not function exclusively within the confines of the body. Through the retina of the eye, for example, and the nerves that receive and convey sensory perceptions of the world, the brain operates outside the skull, confirming and interacting with external events, as well as those that occur inside the body. (Other

16

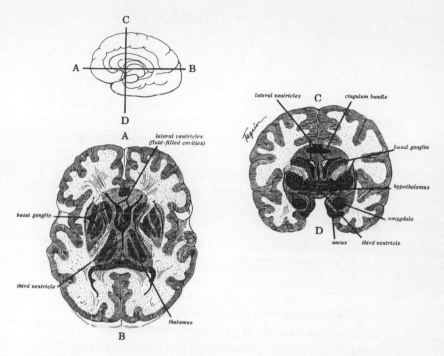

FIG. 5. Cerebrum: (*left*) horizontal section and (*right*) coronal section. Horizontal (*A–B*) and coronal (*C–D*) section of brain hemispheres allows us to inspect some details of deeper limbic brain structures. These limbic areas are shaded in the diagrams.

examples of the brain functioning outside the body would include the senses of smell, hearing, and touch.)

Our human brain is unique in another way: it has the capacity, after perceiving these events, to store them for future reference in its own tissue. This process, of course, is what we call memory, and it is an essential part of learning, for past experiences of all kinds play an important role in determining an individual's reaction to current environmental stimuli. To put it another way, past environment in the form of memory determines to a great extent how we react to our present environment, but memory itself is actually incorporated in brain

17

tissue, and thus information retrieval is obviously a brain process.

Our past environment, once it is past, is no longer simply a sociological phenomenon. It is embedded in our brain, and its use is dependent on the function or malfunction of brain tissue. Modern study of memory function, with magnetic resonance imaging (MRI) and positron emission tomography (PET) scanning observing short-term working memory, shows that a number of different areas of the brain may be involved with different kinds of memory. These will be discussed in more detail in the next chapter. However, vital memory is closely associated with the emotional brain.

In fact, major parts of the memory circuit are in the same anatomical location as the emotional brain. We know that these areas are important for memory because of what happens when they are damaged. If, for example, both hippocampi are injured, a patient may be unable to remember what happens from one minute to the next. If someone says "good morning" to him and then moves out of his sight for more than thirty seconds, the patient will not be able to remember seeing or speaking to the other person when she steps in front of him again. Memories from before the time of injury may remain intact, but the inability to retain recent memory will produce significant deterioration in mental abilities.

In contrast, lesions or damage to the thalamus may cause profound deficits in the entire memory relationship to the world. The whole personality structure may be involved in such a memory loss, with distressing changes in behavior. For example, a forty-three-year-old accountant who suffered a severe brain hemorrhage became disoriented as to time, place, and person. He was awake, alert, and able to see and follow objects. He could move both his hands and his feet. However, he retained only one item out of this cultural past. He kept repeating over and over again the phrase "the fastest gun in the West," which was all that he remembered. He did not recognize his own wife and children when they came to visit him. To their pathetic attempts to remind him who they were, he could only reply, "the fastest gun in the West, the fastest gun in the West."

Another aspect of memory is the ability to retain and follow cultural rules governing behavior. The rules for urination, for example, are culturally determined and rigidly controlled and enforced. We learn these rules when we are young and follow them explicitly thereafter. Yet a lesion in the brain is able to destroy even this kind of important memory.

A case that illustrates this point is that of a sixty-two-year-old retired mill worker who suffered intractable pain resulting from cancer. Medication did not help him, and the only way to control his pain was to make a destructive lesion in the limbic part of his frontal lobe. After he recovered from the operation, he went back to his normal routine as if nothing had happened. He said that he felt well, and he insisted that he and his wife go to see a movie. He dressed himself perfectly, then walked with his wife from their house to the theater. His conversation was witty and polite. About halfway there, however, he said, "excuse me," and in full view of oncoming traffic and pedestrians he urinated in the street! The man's vital memory regarding the rules of urination had been lost.

Lest you think that memory is a uniquely human characteristic (although some aspects of human memory are quite different and distinct in complexity and sophistication from memory of other animals), it really isn't. The basic elements of memory, its crucial importance in learning, and its close association with the limbic or emotional brain are very similar in a number of animal species. That's why it is so important to understand the basic brain anatomy of the memory system that we humans, crocodiles, and many other species share in common.

That information helps to explain why memories associated with certain odors, or with emotionally charged stimuli, are so easily learned and so hard to forget. It also should give us a little humility about our wonderful brain with its exceptional memory capacity. In fact, some animals with a more highly developed nose or emotional brain may have a memory capacity that exceeds our own (in certain limited ways). Therefore, I would advise you to not look down on animals with a highly developed nose or limbic (emotional) brain, and the memory functions and the conditioned reflexes they subserve. Some of those species have a much longer and more successful history of survival than we do!

As you go through the following chapters you should compare the kind of memory difficulties you're having with the memory problems that occur when vital memory is impaired. For the most part, I'm sure, you'll conclude that your memory problems are less serious than the ones I discuss. You know the way to the store, for example, and you don't walk carelessly into traffic. It is losses of vital memory such as these which cause elderly people to lose their orientation. Relatives worry that they'll go outside and try to cross in the middle of busy streets or against stoplights and get hurt or killed. These "wanderers" fill many of the places in nursing homes in the United States.

I'd also like you to remember, however, that even when people get to this stage of losing vital memory — when it is decided they are beyond all hope and they're committed to an institution — it may not be the end of the road for them. The sad fact is that many so-called wanderers have brain or bodily disease that affects brain function. But it is sometimes the case that their loss of vital memory, once its cause is discovered, is not only treatable but also completely reversible. Miracle cures are not required; specific therapies are available that can be used successfully to bring people back to live normal lives, therapies that recoup lost vital memory when symptoms are caused by one of the treatable forms of brain injury or disease.

Never just assume that if memory goes, it is gone forever.

Literally scores of different conditions can result in a person's losing all or part of vital memory, conditions that are treatable and reversible. The important point to remember is that the problem or condition causing memory loss has to be identified. A rational course of treatment or prevention cannot begin until the problem has been precisely identified. If the problem is treatable, much can be done. And keep in mind, new information and better treatments are being developed every year.

If you're wondering if you or someone else has a reversible memory loss problem, one that is susceptible to some of the newer treatments, there are a number of ways to improve your chances of a successful outcome. The first step is for an accurate and complete history to be taken in order to provide a clear explanation of the symptoms. When did the memory loss begin? Is the memory loss selective — that is, can the person no longer remember the name of an old friend but still recognize people whom he or she comes in contact with every day? Or is it just the opposite: do ancient memories remain while the person has trouble with recent memory? Memory is like a complex machine with many intricate components. If there's a malfunction, it helps greatly to know just which part isn't working.

To that end, it's important that you understand more about memory so that if and when you do talk with someone about fixing a problem, you'll be able to comprehend better what the problem is. This book will help you understand memory loss and guide you to find the kind of help you need for your specific difficulty. In the next chapters we take a brief look at the memory process and how to test for a memory problem before we discuss ways of diagnosing and reversing memory loss.

2

The Memory Process

ONE OF THE REASONS it's so difficult to understand memory — its mechanisms and what influences it most — is the fact that it is a brain function that is hidden from view. It can't be studied and analyzed, for example, the way we might study how our hands move. Furthermore, the experts who study memory, behavioral neurologists and neuropsychologists, use slightly different terms to describe the same mechanisms, so the vocabulary is confusing.

Behavioral neurologists, for instance, often talk about the memory process, by which they mean ways of holding information that exceeds an individual's attention span. Memories are physically encoded in the chemistry of brain tissue, forming what are known as *engrams*. According to behavioral neurologists, encoding means converting environmental cues into physical, anatomical changes. They talk about "chunking" — how the brain divides complex information so that it can be more easily assimilated and understood — and "linking" — relating environment, all the cues that surround the information that is memorized, to emotions.

Neuropsychologists, by contrast, describe the memory process somewhat differently. They claim that a memory trace is laid down in the brain, and whether it is a shallow trace that is easily forgotten or a deep trace that the mind holds long afterward is related to the emotional content or other related environmental stimuli and the intensity of those stimuli.

How Doctors Examine the Memory Process

The brain is not a *tabula rasa,* or clean slate, written on by experience. It is a mechanism with inherent capacities for locomotion; autonomic regulation of breathing, heart rate, and blood pressure; and certain feeding abilities, along with genetically acquired traits that manifest themselves as the central nervous system develops. These inherent abilities of the nervous system are molded and shaped by the environment, however, and the molding and shaping — which is a type of learning — are an important aspect of memory. Once memories are formed, they are incorporated into brain structure by physicochemical alterations.

It is impossible to dissociate the brain from its surroundings after environmental stimuli have been laid down as memories in various parts of the brain tissue. This process involves the electrical transmissions from one nerve cell to another in the brain and the chemical changes that take place within and around brain cells. These changes are mediated by special kinds of chemicals called neurotransmitters.

Doctors have learned about the relationship of memory to specific portions of the brain by examining the brains of patients who have died from diseases that produce memory loss. Post-mortem examinations of persons with Korsakoff's psychosis, for example, which is associated with alcoholism and vitamin B-1 deficiency, have shown that the loss of recent memory caused by the disease is related to a lesion in the thalamus. We also know from examining the brains of people who have had loss of recent memory caused by brain injury, or in some cases by symmetrical brain strokes or cerebral infarctions, that lesions of the temporal lobes, especially in the inner anterior portion, may produce such memory loss if the lesions occur on both sides of the brain. One famous case confirmed this discovery. When a neurosurgeon took out both inner anterior portions of the temporal lobes to treat epilepsy, he cured the epilepsy but produced a dramatic loss of recent memory which did not improve.

New diagnostic technologies (for example, magnetic resonance imaging and positron emission tomography [PET] scanning, discussed further below) that have become popular in the last few years have led to new ways of classifying memory. Previously, clinical scientists classified memory only as either short-term or long-term. Now, however, some clinicians believe that memory is composed of several independent but interacting systems, including what they call "episodic memory" and "semantic memory." Episodic memory is defined as the recollection of personal events and semantic memory as the recollection of general knowledge.

The previous method for determining the location of memory sites in the brain developed almost accidentally. After patients with a brain injury or disease died, scientists would try to correlate the parts of memory that were lost with the parts of the brain that were destroyed. Using some of the newer technologies, it's now possible to localize memory sites during life, correlating memory functions with changes in blood flow in the brain. The remarkable thing that scientists have discovered is that more parts of the brain are involved in the memory process than were previously realized. For example, the results of PET scans focused on regional blood flow indicate that networks of brain regions service both episodic and semantic memory.

The tests that we described above were used on normal people, but we can still use magnetic resonance scanning to help us understand memory localization even when the brain has been damaged by tumors, strokes, or injury. For example, Dr. K. Yasuda and his colleagues in Japan recently reported the case of a middle-aged woman who developed a brain tumor near the base of her brain. She had brain surgery and radiation treatment, and afterwards a magnetic resonance scan showed some destruction in her left and right temporal lobes and in her right frontal lobe. The woman also had mild neurological deficits. As far as her memory was concerned, her episodic memory (autobiographical information) remained almost normal. However, her semantic memory (her recollection of public events, historical figures, cultural items, and technical terms related to her profession) was severely impaired. The physicians who studied her memory with neurological and psychological tests suggested that the bilateral lesions in the anterior middle part of both temporal lobes played a crucial role in causing deficits in her semantic memory. In other words, this is a case of technology helping to define the localization of semantic memory.

On the other hand, studies using magnetic resonance imaging in normal volunteers concluded that the encoding of episodic memories showed a localization in the posterior portion of the temporal lobe. The specific part of the temporal lobe involved in these memories was the posterior part of the hippocampus. These studies did not find a difference between the left and the right sides of the brain as is sometimes seen in anatomical correlates of semantic memory. This means that episodic memory is not necessarily represented on both sides of the brain.

Some psychologists and clinicians use another term, "working memory," to describe an important component of short-term and very short-term memory. They claim, and I would agree with them, that working memory is responsible for the short-term and very short-term storage and "online" manipulation of information necessary for higher brain functions, such as language, planning, and problem solving.

Traditionally, working memory has been divided into two types of processes: executive control (that is, governing the encoding, manipulation, and retrieval of information in working memory) and active maintenance (that is, keeping information available online). Some scientists have proposed that these two types of processes may be served by distinct brain structures: the prefrontal cortex, related chiefly to the executive control processes, and the more posterior regions of the brain, related to memory storage.

The definition of the parts of the brain involved in working memory varies to some extent according to the kind of patient or subject being tested, the kind of instrument used in the tests, and the functions of the brain that are included in each definition. A number of unexpected results have occurred in attempts to find the locations of working memory in the brain. For example, studies of working memory using magnetic resonance imaging in normal volunteers indicate that the prefrontal cortex, along with the parietal cortex, plays a role in active maintenance of working memory. Working memory involving visual images activates several areas in the occipital (visual) cortex as well as the prefrontal region. Separate working memory areas in the prefrontal cortex have been identified for memory maintenance of objects, faces, and patterns. Spatial working memory usually activates the middle part of the frontal cortex on the right side. The cingulate gyrus was activated by nonspatial working memory tasks, especially in the left hemisphere.

In other studies of the verbal aspects of working memory localization using PET scanning, it was found that the lateral prefrontal cortex played an important role in both verbal and nonverbal memory. However, only the inferior part of the left frontal lobe was involved in strictly verbal memory.

The more complicated working memory tasks become, the greater the area of brain necessary for successfully carrying out the working memory task. Thus, additional areas of the frontal lobe near the midline as well as parts of a parietal lobe are activated on magnetic resonance imaging studies of more complex memory tasks. Even studies involving verbal working memory may involve not only attention but also executive function and other short-term memory processes.

It is obvious to me that psychologists and some other memory clinicians are trying to correlate complicated memory functions with parts of the brain activated by these memory activities as recorded by PET and magnetic resonance imaging scans. What is not so obvious is that the brain functions being studied are not pure memory. Working memory by its very definition involves other functions associated with, but not intrinsic to, the memory process.

The studies of these complicated memory processes are important as an investigative and research tool. They may, in the future, become useful clinical tools. Today they are certainly used extensively by some psychologists and researchers who are interested in studying memory. The processes are presented here so that you can appreciate some of the newer techniques used to define memory. However, for our purposes, I think that there is a simpler way to understand the memory process, a way that is more useful for the diagnosis and treatment of memory disorders.

When I look at the memory process, I am influenced by the hundreds of patients that I have seen with memory difficulties. And, from my point of view, this influence is more important than the newer concepts of the psychologists or the memory researchers in actually diagnosing and treating patients.

I agree with the notion of a holistic environmental record, an integrated mixture of data from our senses of vision, hearing, taste, smell, and touch to form an image, a word, a number, or even an idea or concept. But whether our brains take in these records or not depends on our concentration — our focus of attention. If you are distracted, it is less likely that such a record will enter your brain. If it does, but your concentration is not intense, the event will produce either a shallow memory trace or a weak engram not stored very securely and probably soon forgotten.

It has been argued by some that every event in our lives is indelibly etched in our brains at one level or another. To support this claim some investigators have shown that under hypnosis a subject can remember details of a crime, for example, that he or she was not aware of — say, the license plate number or appearance of the getaway car. But the fact is that memory is selective, and not every detail is remembered.

I do agree that certain things can rivet the attention and make it more likely that a strong memory will be retained. If an event is emotionally charged — that is, if it is associated with anger or fear — or if it is connected with a strong stimulus such as a very pleasant or unpleasant odor or taste, or a loud noise, or a striking visual image, it is more likely to be retained for a long period of time in our memory banks.

There is a good reason why such stimuli are remembered. The limbic or emotional portion of the brain, particularly the part of the limbic brain where the perception of smell is centered, is closely related to the memory circuits in the temporal lobes, the fore part of the brain on either side to the level of the ears. When this part of the brain is activated, the electrochemical mechanisms associated with memory are likely to be more intense, and the memory traces tend to be more enduring.

Memory Aids

For your information, just so you'll be aware of what they are and how they work, I'll briefly explain some memory aids. Many books are available which teach you how to have a better memory for lists of items or people's names, and the following description is not meant to be all-inclusive or complete.

Books that teach you how to have a better memory often

take advantage of linking as a factor in the memory process. In fact, the field of mnemonics, linking or associating new data to be remembered with images or other known information, is well recognized by psychologists.

Associating objects to be remembered with images is one of the easiest forms of memory building. Here's how it works. If, for example, you're going to the grocery store and want to buy peanut butter, jelly, lettuce, salad dressing, onions, bread, and syrup, you can remember the items on your list by linking them with "pegs" that you've previously memorized, which represent numbers from one to ten. If your first peg is, for example, a shoe and the first item on your list is peanut butter, you might imagine peanut butter spread all over a shoe. In a similar fashion you would then form separate and unusual images for each item you need to remember. Another method of linking is called acronym building. As you know, an acronym is a word that is formed from the first letters of words, such as ASAP for "as soon as possible," or ZIP code for "zone improvement plan" code. Pegs and acronyms are the easiest memory aids to learn to use, and the simplest. If you have trouble remembering people's names or items on shopping lists, I encourage you to read one of the many excellent books on memory improvement at your bookstore or library.

Concentration, Hypnosis, and Sleep

The key to making any memory system work is concentration, which opens the mind to environmental cues and other information. It is a seeming paradox that persons in a state of hypnosis can get and learn new information and keep it after they have come out of the hypnotic state. This phenomenon is called posthypnotic suggestion. Hypnosis is itself a form of hyperconcentration in which extraneous stimuli have been excluded; it is very different from sleep, and claims that certain methods allow learning while sleeping are unfounded. Once an individual has gone through the rapid eye movement stage into the deeper stages of sleep, the chance of meaningful stimuli reaching the memory circuits and being remembered is slight because concentration and attention-focusing mechanisms are very diminished.

To sum up, I don't believe people in deep stages of sleep can remember information from their surroundings. They are simply unable to focus their attention or concentrate enough to enable most environmental cues to enter the brain in any meaningful way.

Memory Storage

Once memories are encoded, they are stored in the brain. The storage process, according to behavioral neurologists, has two mechanisms: consolidation, that is, the transferring of new information into permanent storage in the brain; and organization and reassemblage of memories when they're called on by ongoing activity or the will of the individual.

I call this whole mechanism of storage the memory bank. Although it is often spoken of as having its locus in a single spot in the brain, the memory bank is actually distributed among a number of parts. Visual memories, for example, are located near the visual centers of the brain, auditory memories near the hearing centers of the brain, and so on. Thus, specific brain injuries or strokes in the visual centers can impair visual memories without causing much reduction of vital memory. Brain injuries or diseases of the memory bank system which do impair or obliterate vital memory must be very extensive in both hemispheres of the brain or very deep within the brain, or both. Fortunately, such damage is uncommon.

Memory Retrieval

The last stage of the memory process is memory retrieval, which involves not only scanning for memories but also their reassemblage or reconstitution in our minds. There are two distinct aspects of memory retrieval. The first is an almost instantaneous process that occurs when challenges to our safety arise. If someone throws something at us, for example, we will immediately duck out of the way — a behavior we may not have practiced in many years, since the days we took part in snowball fights, but the memory is still there. The point is, we don't just stand there and allow ourselves to be hit.

The second, more complicated mechanism involves the willed retrieval of memories. As our memory banks become filled with a catalogue of various memories, those engrams we haven't used in a long time may be difficult to retrieve. I'm sure you've had the same experience I've had of trying to recall the name of someone I haven't seen in years, or even perhaps only a few months. It can elude me so completely that I finally give up and stop thinking about it. Then, a few minutes to a few hours later, the name will pop into my head. The retrieval mechanism was still working; it just took a while to be effective.

One of the reasons it is important for someone giving a speech to practice it before the actual delivery, even when it's meant to be rather extemporaneous, is that the act of practicing allows the person to refurbish the memories that surround the subject of the speech. It puts the memory bank on notice that those memories should be close to the surface for retrieval.

The experience of a well-known doctor and friend of mine illustrates a good example of how retrieval works — and sometimes doesn't work. When he was active and presenting papers at scientific meetings, my friend was well prepared to answer questions on any related topic posed to him by his audience, and he did so accurately and quickly. However, after he retired from academic life and was no longer speaking to his colleagues on a daily basis, or preparing to give papers at scientific meetings, his responses were quite different.

On one occasion when, at the last minute, he was asked to stand in at a medical conference, he was quite embarrassed to find that he could not even recall the name of the moderator — even though the worthy man had at one time worked for him as one of his residents in a hospital! The fact is that once this brain scientist had withdrawn from the scientific world, his contacts were no longer doctors and scientists. It's not surprising that without continual practice and review of scientific matters, and contact with the people he had worked with, his retrieval process on those subjects wasn't as efficient as it had been.

The more universes that we are involved in, the more difficult it is to switch from one to the other without preparation. For example, I knew a nurse named Shelley who worked at two different hospitals. While Shelley was working at the first hospital, she could of course identify her co-workers by name without hesitation. However, if a doctor from the second hospital came by chance to the first while Shelley was there, she had great difficulty in recognizing him. Is such behavior abnormal or evidence of some major brain or memory problem? Usually not. In and of itself, without other and potentially more serious problems, I would say that it is a relatively common occurrence.

The moral to these stories is, don't become impatient with yourself when the retrieval process takes longer than you'd like. If you have a large memory bank with a substantial catalogue of memories, don't expect all of them to pop to the surface without some effort on your part to concentrate and make the memories you need available.

Different Kinds of Memory:
Art, Music, Athletic Ability

Up to this point in our discussion of the mechanisms of memory we've been focusing on memories related to language and words. But of course there are a number of different kinds of memory, just as there are different kinds of intelligence. People who play musical instruments are well aware of their ability to memorize pieces of music, retaining memories that have little to do with words and in fact are probably in a different hemisphere of the brain.

In one of its forms, Alzheimer's disease severely affects verbal abilities and verbal memories. I remember seeing a fifty-two-year-old insurance salesman from Denver whose career was interrupted by rapidly progressing Alzheimer's. Much of his vital memory was lost, and he almost had to be led around by his wife. A CAT scan showed that he had a very large loss of tissue, particularly in the speech centers in the left, or dominant, hemisphere of his brain. But just looking at the man's x rays and assessing his speech abilities gave a misleading evaluation of his overall potential. When he was seated at the piano, for example, he could still give a creditable rendition of some difficult pieces of both classical and popular music. His musical ability was obviously not impaired.

Similarly, artistic abilities and memories can be preserved even though verbal memory is quite deficient. I would like to see a controlled experiment done in nursing homes in the United States, many of which have large populations of Alzheimer's victims with severe loss of verbal memory. The walls of the rooms of Alzheimer's patients would be adorned with colorful paintings or perhaps simply soothing colors, while speakers piped in relaxing or stimulating music, depending on what response was desired. The study would compare patients given visual and auditory (artistic and musical) stimulation with similar patients who were not to see if the former patients required as much medication, if they were as uncomfortable, and if their general level of function deteriorated as quickly, including their ability to attend to their basic physical needs. My guess is that the nursing home patients who had a more stimulating environment would require less medication.

Muscular and even athletic abilities have a memory component to them. If an athlete in a competitive sport, particularly one facing an adversary, has a deterioration in memory of the responses required to counteract his or her opponent, performance deteriorates. Produced by conditioned responses, habits only become habitual because of the memory process. When muscular coordination or motor habits are interfered with because of a loss of memory, performance will deteriorate.

I myself think that the motor or performance habits are extremely susceptible to memory loss, and that such deterioration occurs in participants in athletic contests even when their strength and reflex speed seem to be unimpaired. Athletic memories have such immediacy that only a slight deterioration may result in a large decrease in performance.

New Medical Instruments and Their Uses

New instruments have recently been developed which help doctors measure various abnormalities of the brain and correlate them with brain activity and memory. One such instrument is a computerized brain wave machine that records and maps brain waves on a replica of the head. CAT (computerized axial tomography) scans of the brain — a type of x ray which lets us examine the brain tissue as well as the surrounding bone — allow us to see the anatomical structure of the brain and its abnormalities. Using this technique we have been able to learn much more about how brain structures work, and we are now able to correlate destructive changes with losses of recent memory.

Yet another tool available to brain researchers and clinicians is magnetic resonance imaging. This tool, like the CAT scan, allows us to safely and quickly visualize the anatomical structures of the brain. Compared to CAT scanning, with this technique brain structures are visualized more precisely and realistically.

Magnetic resonance imaging works by applying a powerful electromagnetic field to the head. Since the most common magnetic nucleus in the body is that of hydrogen (a proton), whose distribution is similar to that of water, the intense external magnetic field applied to the head causes all the protons in the head to become aligned with this external magnetic field. As the magnetic field alternates rapidly, the direction of the nuclear spins will change. The resulting data are used to develop images reflecting tissue composition in three dimensions.

Still more recently, we've been able to look at the function of the brain tissue in three dimensions by taking what are known as tomographic sections after a patient has been injected with a radioactive isotope. The most accurate (and most expensive) method of doing this is called positron emission tomography, or PET scanning. PET scans involve the use of positron emitting isotopes produced by a cyclotron. (A cyclotron is a machine that accelerates particles in a magnetic field.) The cyclotron, in turn, is used in conjunction with radiation detection devices equipped with computers.

Single photon emission computer tomography (SPECT) can be accomplished with an imaging device that does not require a cyclotron, which is an advantage because it's a lot less expensive than PET scanning. However, the potential for this kind of imaging to provide quantitative information is less than that of PET scans, and the spatial resolution is also lower.

Positron emission tomography gives us the opportunity to produce a dynamic picture of changes in brain function. Often, PET scans yield color intensity pictures, in which areas of increased metabolism appear in red and less active portions are in blue or purple.

As I stated above, not only are PET scans used to detect abnormalities in people with brain problems, but they also give us fascinating insights into some aspects of brain function in normal volunteer subjects. When an individual tested by such a technique is told, for example, to concentrate visually, that is, to look at a particular object, the visual cortex in the back of the brain "lights up." When the subject is asked to listen to a particular sound, the auditory centers in the inner part of the temporal lobes light up. When the individual is given a task requiring substantial thinking, portions of the frontal lobes light up. And when a subject is asked to remember a visual object, metabolism increases not only in the visual cortex but also in portions of the temporal lobes — those parts that we've already indicated to be important in memory function. Such scans create a rather striking picture of at least some memory functions, giving us hope that we may be able to trace certain kinds of brain function more accurately with similar techniques.

More recently, magnetic resonance imaging has been refined and improved to produce a technique called functional magnetic resonance imaging. This new technique produces the images of activated brain regions (stimulated by vision, sound, or other environmental cues) by detecting the indirect effects of neural activity on local blood volume, flow, and oxygen saturation. The use of functional magnetic resonance imaging at least partially competes with positron emission tomography. However, it has the advantage of being noninvasive, and it has better spatial and temporal resolution.

Functional magnetic resonance imaging is different from regular magnetic resonance imaging in that instead of relying on one slice of the brain, this technique uses multi-slice, echo-planar images. It does not completely replace PET scans, however, because PET scans measure aspects of brain function that cannot be tested by magnetic resonance imaging.

The new brain imaging techniques, functional magnetic resonance scans, PET scans, and SPECT scans, together create a fantastic new approach to help us understand how the brain works. They give us the opportunity to correlate function with structure in the living brain, truly a milestone in the history of medicine. Furthermore, the tests are benign, so that they can be carried out in normal volunteers. In the next few years, as scientists complete the mapping of all the normal brain functions, I believe we will have a much better chance for the very early diagnosis and improved treatment of brain abnormalities when they do occur.

3

Memory Testing

WHAT KINDS of memory loss are serious enough for you to consult a neurologist about? What memory symptoms should you look for in yourself or your relatives which are of real concern? The short answer is that any memory problem that is persistent or severe enough to cause you to worry about it should send you to your doctor. Even if it proves to be inconsequential, it's worth your while to know that it isn't serious, and finding that out should shield you from needless anxiety and the secondary depression that can make a trivial memory problem into a disabling symptom.

But aren't some memory symptoms more important than others, symptoms that demand more medical attention and formal memory testing? Yes, but they vary in degree and seriousness. For example, if someone is able to drive the same route every day for years without difficulty and suddenly begins to get lost, that's a sign that formal memory testing and neurological or neuropsychological testing should be done. If someone you know tells the same story over and over again, and does so even after telling the story less than an hour before, memory testing is mandatory. If someone has a pattern of forgetfulness which is progressive and disabling to the point that memory loss interferes with job performance or basic functioning, memory testing is imperative.

Mind you, the situations I've described do not involve forgetting things like items on a shopping list, where you put your keys, or someone's name. But as I've said, any memory symptoms that cause you anxiety should be looked into, to prevent unnecessary worry and worsening of the symptoms. Whether it is done by a neurologist or a neuropsychologist, memory testing is the most important initial diagnostic step to separate serious complaints from trivial ones.

Before I describe specific memory tests, it is useful to point out that the memory abilities each of us is born with, or ultimately develops, differ. Some of us have better musical memory, or artistic memory, or athletic memory. Some of us have a very fine mathematical or scientific memory, whereas others are especially endowed with good verbal memory. Regardless of what the ability is, as a rule the more a memory function is used, the better preserved it will be as we grow older — as long as the memory function in the brain is not weakened by brain injury or brain disease.

As we grow older, we generally experience what is known as benign memory loss, which means, for one thing, that many of us have difficulty remembering individuals' names. Several studies have indicated that older people have difficulty in short-term learning and with short-term memory, but these problems don't occur in everyone. Studies reviewed by Robert Katzman and Robert D. Terry, for example, showed that fourteen people who had taken a test of mental efficiency and were then retested thirty-five years later, when they were between sixty and seventy-four years old, had unchanged or even slightly improved vocabulary scores. Their overall learning scores, however, decreased from an average of seventeen to an average of thirteen (on a scale of zero to twenty), and the results of retention tests declined from eighteen to thirteen over the thirty-five-year period. But there were wide differences among subjects, and those who were not hypertensive exhibited no decline in their memory scores over a ten-year period.

One reason older people may not do as well as younger ones on memory tests is that they may not have been taught to use various mnemonic techniques in new learning. What one is really measuring, then, is a cultural rather than a physiological phenomenon of the brain.

Of course, memory is an important part of all new learning. In order to find out whether a person's memory is functioning at optimal level it is necessary to perform tests, both simple and elaborate, of learning and memory abilities. Typically, either a psychologist or a neuropsychologist is the trained medical professional who does such testing. I won't include an entire test here since it would be far too long and detailed for you to use. But I will explain what is usually tested for, and why, so that you'll understand the importance of these tests in determining the cause of reversible memory loss.

Auditory and Visual Testing

One of the most common ways in which a neuropsychologist tests memory is to see how rapidly a given subject can learn visual or auditory information. Data are presented, for example, in the form of cards showing words or pictures. The subject is given a limited period of time to study these cards and is then asked to recall the information after one, two, or three repetitions.

Auditory learning is tested in the same way, with verbal instructions presented regarding words, phrases, or ideas. After suitable delays, and at times with repetitions and cues, the subject is asked to repeat the information in either writing or speech. These tests evaluate not only a person's visual and auditory memory but also other aspects of intelligence and language function.

A Neurological Memory Test

As a neurologist, I usually divide memory testing into three parts to correspond with the three major aspects of memory: immediate recall, recent memory, and ancient (or remote) memory.

When I test immediate recall I'm not only testing immediate memory but also an individual's attention span. For example, I will give someone seven numbers — 5, 6, 8, 4, 3, 2, 7 — and ask the person to repeat them. Then I will give the same individual five numbers and have the person repeat those in reverse order. Keep in mind that people with severe deficiencies in recent-memory ability can still repeat numbers or phrases like "no ifs, ands, or buts" if their attention spans are of normal duration.

Testing of recent memory gives a more penetrating assessment of memory abilities. Here I ask the subject to remember the names of three or four unrelated objects, such as a table, a flower, and a book, but I don't allow the person being tested to keep repeating the list over and over in his or her mind. If I did that I wouldn't be testing recent memory; I'd be back at immediate memory or immediate recall. What I do is intersperse my questions about the list items with a number of other questions which focus attention on another topic. For example, I give various instructions, I ask mathematical questions, I ask the subject to interpret proverbs, I ask geographical questions, and I make the questions difficult enough so that the person's mind cannot revert to the original words that are supposed to be remembered. Then, after three and a half to four minutes, I ask the subject to repeat the three or four words in the same sequence I gave them. The point of this test of recent memory is that it demands that a person be able to hold information exceeding his or her attention span for the words to be remembered.

41

Ancient memory testing is somewhat trickier. At one time I used to test ancient memory by asking patients questions about geography: for example, What states border Massachusetts? Now, however, if I test persons under the age of thirty-five, they probably won't be able to tell me — not because of their deficient memories but rather because of their deficient education, since geography is rarely taught in our public school systems anymore.

Because presidents and often past presidents are figures in the news, and because most people at one time or another watch television news, I usually test ancient or remote memory by having the subject give me the name of the current president followed by those of preceding presidents. Again, older patients seem to do better on this test than younger ones, who complain, "Well, of course, I wasn't alive when Truman or Eisenhower was president." What they're really telling me is that American history was not taught effectively in their schools.

Ancient memory is best tested through those memories we all have in common. It is very difficult to get a valid test of remote memory by asking people about the events of their private lives without independent verification from relatives — and even so, the information gathered in this way may be misleading since "normal" family members can have widely differing views on how a specific event or story unfolded. Also, individuals with severe damage to the inner parts of both anterior temporal lobes, who have great difficulty with recent memory and in learning new information, also make up stories. If you ask them about events in their private lives in order to test remote memory, they may give a very complete account that is nevertheless absolutely false.

Such was the case with George, a thirty-eight-year-old social science teacher at a Boston high school, who had a benign tumor in the center of his brain. By benign I mean that it was not cancerous, it did not metastasize, and it didn't invade the surrounding brain, but it produced symptoms because it pressed on sensitive areas of the brain. As the tumor grew larger it could not be treated with deep x-ray therapy alone, and therefore as much of it as possible had to be removed surgically.

George had severe loss of recent memory before the operation, and although the tumor was removed almost in its entirety, it had already caused enough damage to central brain structures that his loss of recent memory persisted in the postoperative period. If I went to see him in his room, for example, he would talk to me quite pleasantly. But if I were called away for a minute or two and then came back into the room, he would not remember that he had just seen me. He would greet me all over again as though it were a completely new conversation, and he would swear that he had never seen me before. He was absolutely convinced that he was telling the truth.

In addition, George told me about his life experiences in the most exaggerated terms. Rather than a high school teacher, he implied he was a famous college professor and lecturer (perhaps his secret ambition); he also said he was married and had four lovely children. Our investigations failed to disclose that he had ever been married or had any children.

Even though he described his past life in great detail, my conversation with his elderly parents failed to substantiate any of his claims. He was, in fact, demonstrating the symptoms of confabulation. This false reporting of remote memory occurs in many diseases that involve the center of the brain, in an area called the thalamus and hypothalamus. Not only tumors but also hemorrhages, strokes, and nutritional deficiencies such as an insufficient amount of thiamine, or vitamin B-1, in the diet (a deficiency associated with alcohol abuse) often produce this syndrome. George wasn't purposefully trying to deceive me or anyone else. But because of his condition, he remembered his life as having been very different from what it was, and far more successful. With the removal of the tumor and subsequent deep x-ray treatments, however, he gradually regained some of his memory abilities, although his recollection of much of his childhood and school years did not return.

To sum up, since neurologists and neuropsychologists can't rely on personal memories in testing remote-memory ability, they will carry out tests for information that should have been learned in school or that is part of our historical or political heritage.

Let me assure you first that if your immediate recall, recent memory, and remote memory are normal, it is unlikely that you have anything to worry about as far as vital memory functions are concerned. Also, if you do have some problems in memory testing, it doesn't necessarily mean you are suffering from an incurable brain disease. In fact, it may mean that you simply need to have a good medical and neurological assessment. There are many treatable causes of memory loss, and such loss can be promptly reversed with effective therapy, which I will describe in later chapters.

As we look at examples of memory problems in various persons, you will see that the pattern of memory loss in each is significant and that these different patterns can be discovered and diagnosed by various mental status and psychological tests. Individuals who are agitated or depressed may have a variable pattern in their memory tests, as was the case with Gary, forty-three, a restaurant manager who came to see me after he began to forget lists of items he was going to the supermarket to buy.

Gary's memory was so bad, he told me, that he even forgot to kiss his wife when he left for work. His memory tests did show areas of memory lapse, both visual and auditory. Some mistakes in recent memory were made, and some in remote recall. But Gary also had islands of memory proficiency which were outstanding. He would remember the list of objects in the test of recent memory very well on one occasion and not at all on another. He could remember the names of only three presidents on one test occasion, but rattled off the names of seven mayors of Boston in reverse order with ease.

This variable test pattern indicated a disorder like mild depression, not stroke or Alzheimer's, as the cause of Gary's problem, and this problem was eminently treatable. By contrast, Hank, a fifty-one-year-old department store salesman, wasn't himself at all concerned about memory loss; it was his relatives who insisted he come to see me. They complained that he kept telling the same old stories to them over and over, sometimes after only fifteen-minute intervals. Hank also got so lost when he was driving that they no longer allowed him to be in a car alone.

Memory testing showed that Hank's results were consistent; repeated tests of recent memory showed him to be very deficient. He also had greater difficulty with material presented visually than with verbal information. The test results didn't necessarily mean that Hank's memory deficiencies were untreatable, but they did show that he had a serious problem requiring complete neurological and medical evaluations. In the next chapter we'll look at what these evaluations consist of, and how someone like Hank can be helped.

Before leaving the subject of memory testing, it will be useful to explore a couple of the most recent advances in memory evaluation. These advances appear to be particularly helpful for people who test as normal but who subjectively realize that their memory abilities are reduced.

Patricia, a product manager at a computer company, presents a good case for what new kinds of testing can do. Three years ago, she suffered a head injury in an automobile collision. Prior to that, she never used written records because she could store an incredible number of facts in her memory with complete reliability. After the accident she was initially unconscious but seemed to make a substantial recovery. However, she found that her memory was not good enough for her to continue on in her job.

Patricia underwent a number of different neurological tests, none of which disclosed any serious trouble. She also had a complete battery of psychometric tests that placed her in the normal range. Nevertheless, she herself knew that she was not normal and that her memory functions were deficient. To try to reach a more accurate diagnosis her doctors referred her to a firm called Cognitive Diagnostics, Inc. This company recently added another dimension to psychometric testing by devising a series of tests to measure the brain's information-processing speed and efficiency by means of a battery of cognitive reaction tasks. The tests render a direct reading of cognitive functioning and threshold capacities across a range of performance variables, including short-term memory, attention, and physical and mental reflexes.

Cognitive reaction time tests were first carried out on completely normal people. This was done to establish the variations that occurred normally. Once the results were confirmed statistically, it was possible to define reliable reaction time changes in Alzheimer's disease, Parkinson's disease, stroke, depression, stress, attention deficit disorder, diabetes, and other conditions that affect the brain.

The company Brain.com developed the "cognometer," which is a self-administered, computerized test battery of perceptual, cognitive, and motor reflexes (reaction times). It is fast to use and appears to be highly accurate. To begin requires an initial tutorial of ten to fifteen minutes, and then it takes about five to ten minutes for patients to establish their baselines. Once an individual's baseline is established, subtle changes in mental status over very short periods of time can be detected and recorded.

This testing technique was designed to work with almost any computer. Computerized test results can usually be delivered in less than ten minutes. The results include measures of simple reaction time (or physical reflexes); inspection time, including perceptual reflexes and thresholds; cognitive choice reaction time; working memory speed and efficiency; working memory capacity, including very short-term memory capacity and the recall speed; and visual-spatial reflexes, among others.

The company has also developed more complex testing techniques that can identify the subtle changes in memory abilities that may be missed by more traditional psychological testing methods. The tests that I have described above are the preliminary self-administered tests that can be used for screening purposes. When they are abnormal this may indicate the need for more complex testing.

In Patricia's case the tests revealed a normal finding in the morning, similar to the results of other psychometric tests. However, because these tests are time sensitive and simple to reduplicate, they were taken by her twice a day for three days, once in the morning and once in the afternoon. The results were striking.

Patricia's morning tests were normal, but her afternoon tests showed that she had trouble focusing her attention, which translated into difficulty in laying down new memories. She also had difficulty in retrieving memories from her memory bank. This was a result of fatigue, a common aftermath of a head injury and one often associated with a post-head-injury depression. Her depression did improve over time, and her symptoms were diminished by repeated memory exercises through a program made available by the company that makes the cognometer.

Incidentally, the cognometer is not the only computerized neuropsychological test. Others appear under their acronym or brand names, such as Microcog, Cantab, and Anam. I prefer the cognometer, however, because at this point it has a more extensive database, it measures a greater range of cognitive performance variables, and it is a faster and more comprehensive memory test.

Testing methods are constantly evolving, along with our understanding of the memory process. This evolution cannot but help us make more accurate diagnoses, which will result in more effective treatments.

PART II

Reversal of Memory Loss

4

Bad Memories and Stress:
The Leading Cause of Memory Loss

IVAN PAVLOV, the Nobel prize-winning Russian physiologist, laid the groundwork for understanding how bad memories can disrupt the memory process when they become incorporated into the brain's menu of powerful conditioned reflexes. Pavlov's experiments with dogs involved the ringing of a bell plus the presentation of a piece of meat to a dog, and measuring the increase in the amount of saliva produced. When the bell ringing and meat presentation were combined often enough, the bell ringing alone, without the meat, was enough to cause the same volume of increased saliva flow — that is, the classic conditioned reflex.

The stories of the following patients illustrate how this powerful brain mechanism can disrupt memory if negative conditioned reflexes are formed, especially if such reflexes are further modified by depression and stress.

I first met Shane Turner some years ago at a party that he gave when he moved into his new house in a suburb outside Boston. He was a born executive — high-energy-level, decisive, intelligent, with a confident and winning personality. At that time, he was opening a number of fast-food franchises, and in fact he was one of the first businessmen in the country to concentrate on theme restaurants. Though in his early thirties, he was already enormously successful and had opened restaurants in major cities throughout the country, including New York, Miami, Phoenix, and Palm Springs.

It surprised me greatly when, a couple of weeks after the party, Shane consulted me in my office about memory loss. My first contacts with him had led me to believe that he had an excellent memory. In fact, he seemed to be able to hold three, or sometimes four, separate trains of thought in his mind at the same time. Not only that, but he could answer a telephone call or greet a new friend and switch to an entirely new line of conversation without missing a beat. But when he sat in my office that particular day, his chief complaint was that he was no longer able to keep even one train of thought in his mind for more than a few seconds.

The interference with Shane's memory function had caused him to lose confidence. He could no longer talk to customers or even senior members of his staff without embarrassing hesitations. Because the success of his restaurant ventures depended almost entirely on his confidence and abilities, concern was starting to set in among his investors. Clearly, this was no time for Shane to lose his cool and allow his business to be wrecked.

The most important part of a medical examination is the taking of a detailed and accurate history. This requires skill on the part of the examiner, and patience. Taking a good history is very time-consuming, but it also can be very rewarding for the patient. When I took Shane's history, I realized that he was certainly no coward or weakling. During World War II, he was a fighter pilot in England. He led his squadron in some of the most dangerous missions of the war and was decorated for bravery. Somehow, however, fighting business battles was different than fighting the Germans. My first impression was that bad conditioned reflexes were responsible for his memory problems. I'll explain at the end of this chapter in detail what conditioned reflexes are, but in brief that means that Shane had "programmed" a certain response, in this case memory loss, based on certain crises occurring.

Before undertaking a treatment program, I had to be certain of my diagnosis. I first performed a complete physical examination, which turned out to be normal. Shane had no disease of his heart, lungs, kidneys, or liver. Then I looked him over neurologically. Part of my neurological examination was an evaluation of his mental status. This was the only part of the examination that was abnormal, as I found that his recent memory was clearly defective.

When I gave Shane three unrelated words to remember for a period of four minutes he couldn't remember one of them. Surprisingly, his memory for recent events in the news was unimpaired. More detailed memory testing showed that he had difficulty in focusing his attention. He was easily distracted, and of course the combination of distraction and the inability to concentrate made it almost impossible for him to encode new memories.

It became obvious to me that this man's bad conditioned reflexes were directly related to the prospect of failure in business. Shane was a man who could face bullets and bombs, but he couldn't face poverty. It turned out that his early childhood was one of intense poverty. Shane's parents had been farmers in Tennessee, and they were not very successful. Whether this was due to poor soil, bad weather conditions, their own lack of skill, or a combination of factors, the result was a nightmare for Shane. Never being warm enough in the winter, always on the verge of hunger, doing backbreaking work in the fields, feeling utter hopelessness when he lost both parents to a flu epidemic — all of these things instilled a deep feeling of fear in Shane that never left him.

On the other hand, fear seemed to have spurred him on to great accomplishments. When Shane was mustered out of the service, he used the money that he had saved to get a first-class education. He even achieved a master's degree from the business school at U.C. Berkeley, and thereafter his rise in the business world was meteoric. It seemed as though nothing could defeat him, except perhaps a sudden change in the economy, something that he had no control over. Then it was the Tennessee winter all over again.

When I explained the origin of the bad conditioned memories to Shane, it was for him as though a light bulb had suddenly gone on inside his head. However, just knowing the origin of his problem did not in itself allow Shane to correct it. He could say over and over again that his feelings were foolish, or that he had to get hold of himself, but that didn't correct his memory problem. It required a definite program to repair the chink in his armor.

Fortunately, Shane had a very understanding and competent wife. The three of us set up a series of memory games that had nothing to do with business, but they were interesting enough to capture Shane's attention. The exercises were repeated three times a day, and each session lasted ninety minutes. The initial memory exercises were simple, and Shane was able to master them easily. Gradually the exercises became more complex. They instilled in him the feeling that he, once again, could control his own memory. The proof was self-evident. He got the right answers, and the more he did the exercises the more confidence he began to feel in his own memory ability.

In between memory exercises, I started him on a program to relax certain parts of his brain. I showed him a brain map that had the sensory and motor areas mapped out. He could see that certain parts of the body had a much bigger representation in the brain than others. For example, the amount of space in the brain devoted to the thumb and fingers is much larger than the amount of space devoted to the arms or shoulders. Similarly, the tongue and lips have a much bigger representation than the scalp. Thus, it made sense to Shane that relaxing the thumbs and fingers would have a more profound effect on relaxing the entire brain than trying, for example, to relax the chest.

I told Shane that it was very important for him to be able to clear his mind of all other thoughts before he began the brain relaxation exercises. We were, in effect, establishing some new conditioned reflexes, and we wanted them to be guided by good memories, not bad ones. I then had him sit in a comfortable chair in a semi-darkened room with his eyes closed. Next I had him concentrate on relaxing just the tip of his right thumb. When that was completely relaxed he concentrated on the part of his thumb closer to his hand. Then I had him do the same thing with the tip of the index finger of his right hand. Sequentially, I had him concentrate on all the other parts of the fingers of his right hand, segment by segment. Then he started the same program with his left hand. (I emphasized to Shane how important it was for him not to go to sleep during the brain relaxation exercises.) Next, he began to concentrate on the various parts of his lips and finally on parts of his tongue. When he finished this program, he was ready to go back to the memory games.

Gradually, I began to introduce small segments of business facts into the memory games. I did this very slowly, however. If this made him uneasy or apprehensive, I would stop the memory games and start him on relaxation exercises.

Fortunately, Shane had some very good lieutenants in his employ. They were able to keep the business afloat for the ten days of Shane's initial treatment. I thought it was very important to separate him completely from his business during the initial treatment phase. It wasn't until he was comfortable with business memories that I felt it was safe for Shane to resume his activities. When he did, the way he took hold of his affairs was quite remarkable. It was as though he had never been ill. He told me that it was as if he had had a broken leg that had suddenly healed — completely. Nevertheless, I told Shane that he had to keep up his exercises, and that the bad conditioned memories were still there. He had to be vigilant to keep them from taking control of his life. The whole secret here was control. When Shane had it, and if he could maintain it, the bad memories would not bother him again.

Not all patients with bad conditioned reflexes and their associated bad memories can be treated as easily and quickly as Shane was. Sometimes memory complaints may be only a small part of a major clinical problem. In such cases the treatment of the memory problem may be an important step in the total treatment of the patient.

Jennifer Bowen had become an important manager with a health care maintenance organization. She'd prided herself on her independence and efficiency, and she was almost distraught when she came to consult me. She had recently been promoted to a new and more demanding position in the company, and she complained that she just couldn't do the work. She couldn't seem to learn new procedures, and she found herself getting more and more confused. On top of that, she began to forget appointments unless she wrote them down in her appointment book. She also found that she kept forgetting where she had put her appointment book, her glasses, and her keys.

Given all the problems she was having, Jennifer was afraid that her boss would demote her, or even fire her. Sooner or later she knew he would find out how much difficulty she was having in adjusting to her new responsibilities.

Just as in the case of Shane, Jennifer's complaints had to be investigated, first and foremost by the taking of a careful and complete history. It turned out that her memory problems were not the only difficulties that she was experiencing. She would also get unexplained episodes of a racing heart, overwhelming feelings of fear, and outright panic, in which she felt that she was going to faint.

When I asked her how long she had had these symptoms,

she said that she was uncertain because they seemed to come on gradually. However, she did say that they had begun before her job promotion. When I questioned her about sources of stress in her life, she readily admitted that there were many. At first, she denied that there had been any change in the stressful situations. Then she was thoughtful for a minute, and said, "You don't mean the lawsuit, do you?"

It seemed that a young woman patient with psychiatric symptoms had been dissatisfied with her treatment at the health maintenance organization. She had complained to a number of people who worked under Jennifer's direction, without any satisfaction. Then one day she'd burst into Jennifer's office and threatened to kill her. Jennifer called security and had the woman ejected. Shortly after that, Jennifer and two other employees of the health maintenance organization were served with a formal complaint that stated that the patient was suing them for three million dollars. The complaint charged them with negligence. It was after she received this summons that Jennifer's symptoms began to appear. This was obviously an important feature of Jennifer's history.

I did a complete physical examination, which showed that Jennifer was quite healthy as far as her heart, lung, liver, kidney, and blood functions were concerned. Her neurological examination was also normal, except, as was the case with Shane, for her mental status evaluation. This showed a dysfunction of her working memory, especially her ability to encode new memories. Her ability to focus her attention and concentrate was abnormal. With this information, we were ready to begin treatment.

Here again, I began by removing her from her job for a period of two weeks, and I started her on some simple memory exercises that were quite unrelated to her work or to the lawsuit. Unfortunately, she was so distracted by the legal threat hanging over her head that she was not able to perform even simple memory exercises. Then I tried the relaxation exercises that had been so helpful in Shane's case. I had to abandon this maneuver, however, because she couldn't concentrate well enough to achieve even simple relaxation of her digits.

It was time to go back to her history and get more information, especially about her lawsuit, since the onset of the lawsuit against her seemed to coincide with the onset of her severe symptoms. It became clear, just as in Shane's case, that loss of control was a pivotal factor in initiating her symptoms. It was also obvious to me that Jennifer liked to control her own destiny. Her struggles to succeed were fueled by her difficult childhood. Her mother had divorced her father, who was an alcoholic, and she had taken Jennifer to live with her. When Jennifer was twelve, her mother died of cancer. In the meantime, her father had married again, and even though he didn't want Jennifer, she had no other place to go. So she went to live with her alcoholic father and her emotionally unsupportive stepmother. The situation was intolerable, and she often imagined herself to be Cinderella. Alas, there was no Prince Charming.

When Jennifer was sixteen she left home. She did menial jobs to support herself and went to night school to get her high school diploma. She started a community college course and finally transferred to a university that had a work-study program. It took her seven years to get her college degree, but she did it.

When she started working for the health maintenance organization, she was in a subservient position, taking orders from others. She didn't like it, but she worked hard and was steadily promoted. Jennifer also took postgraduate courses at night, paid for by her company. Her recent promotions had given her something more than money; they had given her a measure of independence, the freedom to act on her own without interference from anyone. She was finally in control of her own life, or at least so she thought. Then came the sudden lawsuit, and her freedom was taken away from her. It was a classic Catch-22 situation. The more her freedom was threatened, the more her memory functions were impaired, and the worse her job performance became. Of course, the more difficulty that she had with her new job, the more likely she was to lose it and her cherished independence.

I then went into more detail about her lawsuit. A lot of other people have been sued, without losing their memory. Control does not always reside with the plaintiff in a lawsuit. In many cases, the defense has an advantage. What was there about Jennifer's case that made her feel so impotent? Didn't she have a lawyer?

It turned out that she had a lawyer appointed by the insurance company that insured her health maintenance organization, but she didn't trust him. The law firm retained by her health maintenance organization didn't feel that her lawsuit was very important, so they had assigned one of the least experienced lawyers in their office to defend her. She felt that he was incompetent, and she didn't know what to do about it.

I advised Jennifer to call the claims agent for the insurance company that insured her employer, because the claims agent retained the law firm, and a claims agent was someone the law firm would listen to. However, she didn't feel confident enough to do that. So I took the unusual step of calling the claims agent myself. I told the agent that my patient required a better lawyer, not a novice or a beginner in the field. I further explained that the lack of good representation was causing my patient to become sick to the point that she would not be able to cooperate in her defense. Furthermore, I reminded the agent that the insurance company was required to see that their insured was given an adequate defense, and that their failure to do this might leave them vulnerable to subsequent legal action.

The strategy worked. Since the law firm received a lot of work from this particular insurance company, the message that they received from the claims agent got their immediate attention. My patient received a new lawyer the next day — a senior partner who was calm, competent, and in control. More importantly, he gave Jennifer the feeling that she was in control of her own destiny. All of this did not restore her memory abilities, but it did make her accessible to the kind of treatment that I initiated.

Jennifer started simple memory exercises and was able to progress day by day to more complex exercises. She was also able to practice brain relaxation involving larger and larger areas of her cortex. She began to substitute good memories and good conditioned reflexes for the bad ones. Even after the lawsuit against her was dismissed, she still had symptoms of memory difficulty, but they were much less intense and had a shorter duration. After three weeks, she was able to go back to work, although it took several months before she felt that her memory function had returned to normal.

Memory loss may become evident in a number of different ways. Shane and Jennifer had losses of memory related to words and numbers. However, there is also visual memory, related to art and pictures, and memory related to music. There is even memory related to athletic pursuits.

I firmly believe that what frequently ends professional athletic careers isn't purely physical, but rather the fact that professional athletes sometimes lose the good memories associated with good conditioned reflexes as they grow older. Surprisingly, I believe this loss occurs long before they lose muscular strength.

Jimmy K. was a defensive back for a professional football team in the National Football League. He had had three or four very good years and almost made the Pro Bowl one year. Then something happened to him. He didn't seem to react quickly enough to cover wide receivers on opposing teams. He told me that his coach had criticized him for being too mechanical. Jimmy recognized what he had to do but was unsure of his ability to do it.

In taking a careful history, it turned out that Jimmy's problems seemed to begin when his wife left him for another man. He lost control, and he lost confidence in himself. Responses to game situations, which were natural to him before, were now confusing. He couldn't remember what he was supposed to do, and his reactions became slow and uncertain.

I never had the opportunity to help him to condition new memories, either athletic memories or cortical relaxation memories, because Jimmy chose another therapeutic avenue: he started to take a large amount of cocaine. In a short time he became addicted and moved out of the city, and I lost contact with him. Street drugs, particularly cocaine, are never good therapy, especially for the treatment of bad memories, bad conditioned reflexes, and loss of impulse control They are even worse treatment for depression, phobia, and panic response. I include alcohol among such street drugs as cocaine, marijuana, and speed.

Jimmy never made it back into the ranks of professional athletes, but I had better luck in treating Randy, an aspiring concert pianist. Playing the piano is not at all like playing football, yet Randy's complaints, in some peculiar ways, mirrored the complaints of Jimmy. Randy suddenly found that he was unable to play pieces that he had previously been able to play easily. He told me that he would find himself playing the middle of a piece perfectly when suddenly the thought would enter his mind, unbidden, that he wouldn't be able to remember the next measure. Then he would feel as though he couldn't possibly remember the next measure, he would become panicky, and he would have to stop playing. This happened to him during a recital, and the results were catastrophic. By the time he came to me it looked very much as though his promising musical career was at an end.

When I examined Randy, his physical and neurological examinations were completely normal. Even his mental status exam was normal. But the usual mental status examination does not test musical ability or musical memory, so in his case I found my usual bag of tools somewhat limited. However, I've been playing the piano myself for more than sixty years, so I did have a fairly clear idea of what might help another musician, even one considerably more accomplished than I am.

I felt that Randy needed special kinds of memory-conditioned reflexes connected to music, and so I devised for him musical conditioned reflexes that did not involve the pieces that he was practicing. I also tried to initiate cortical relaxation reflexes. After a few weeks, I was disappointed to find that he didn't respond particularly well to my efforts, so I went back to developing more facts from Randy's history. I was particularly interested in things that had happened to him at about the time he began to have difficulty playing the piano.

At first Randy was reluctant to discuss his recent past. It took several sessions to gain his confidence. It turned out that Randy had been informed by his sexual partner that he had tested positive for HIV. Randy was devastated by this news, and he became compulsively fixated on the possibility that he was going to develop AIDS.

The first thing I did was to insist that he be tested, and fortunately, his initial test was negative. Randy understood as I did that one negative test does not necessarily mean that one is free of the disease. However, knowledge is power, and I told him that the more knowledge he had about the disease, how to treat it and how to prevent it, the more control he would have over his own destiny. He gradually overcame some of his early fears and began to read as much information as he could on the subject. It was only after he felt secure in his newly acquired knowledge and in control of himself that he became a fit subject for treatment.

At that point the novel musical conditioned reflex memory treatments and cortical relaxation treatments I devised for Randy began to bear fruit. Eventually we were even able to introduce memory exercises that included musical pieces from his own repertoire into our therapy program, and step by step Randy improved. As he gained confidence in his memory abilities, his pianistic virtuosity began to reassert itself. In several months critics said that he was playing better than ever. Both he and I knew, however, that he would always be susceptible to his bad conditioned memories, initiated by any feelings of loss of control. That is why, even after he felt well, I continued to have him practice his musical memory exercises and his cortical relaxation memory exercises. He had to have a reservoir of good conditioned memories and reflexes to call upon in times of future stress.

Neither Shane's nor Jennifer's cases were particularly serious, but this does not imply that all fears about memory loss are unfounded. I would say, however, that when people fear they are losing their memories because their father or their grandfather had Alzheimer's disease, and think they're experiencing the same kind of memory loss, most of the time they are really suffering from quite a different kind of malady — a negative conditioned reflex. At the beginning of this chapter we described the establishment of powerful conditioned reflexes in the dog. What isn't so well realized is that the establishment of a reflex with its associated memory is actually accomplished more easily in human beings than it is in dogs. Over a period of time, we humans develop thousands of conditioned reflexes and the associated memories that go along with them.

Most conditioning is helpful and is the basis of all new learning. Some conditioning, however, is harmful or negative, particularly when the conditioning is inappropriate. For example, when we have become conditioned to a danger or the threat of a danger, various internal systems in our bodies respond to an impending emergency. Our hearts begin to race, blood vessels constrict, more sugar and oxygen are delivered to vital tissues, and we are prepared to fight or run away.

If the danger is not real, however, if it is something that we just imagine, there will be no one to fight and no place to run. Yet all the internal changes of the body still take place. Those changes can make us feel frightened, full of panic, and filled with somatic complaints of the heart and gut. And the memory of the perceived danger, if repeated often enough, may make us profoundly depressed.

The stress from bad conditioned reflexes, as well as stress induced under experimental conditions, is often associated with increased levels of the steroid hormone cortisol in the body and especially in parts of the brain associated with memory, such as the hippocampus. There is strong reason to believe that cortisol adversely affects not only the function of the hippocampus but also its structure. It is not surprising, therefore, to find that stress and the resulting increase in cortisol levels are often associated with an impairment in certain memory faculties. At times this impairment can be quite severe. This is particularly true if the stress is chronic and results in a dysregulation of the hypothalamic–pituitary–adrenal axis, resulting in chronically raised cortisol levels.

Paradoxically, certain memory functions improve with a reversal of depression when the steroid dehydroepiandrosterone (DHEA) or its sulfate (DHEAS) is administered so as to increase their ratios to plasma cortisol levels. There is also some evidence that classical conditioning as described above can decrease cortisol levels, which may account for some of the memory improvement we saw in Shane and Jennifer.

Most people encounter stress at some point in their lives, but not everyone reacts the same way. People who are depressed and have bad conditioned reflexes (along with the bad memories that are part of those bad conditioned reflexes) are much more susceptible to the effects of stress than healthy individuals. The former group has a longer period of stress anticipation, higher cortisol levels, and more deterioration of memory than healthier individuals. The combination of bad conditioned reflexes with bad memories, stress, and some degree of depression are so intertwined in most people complaining of memory problems that I often regard them as part of the same syndrome. All of these factors have to be taken into account in diagnosing and treating people with this, the most common form of memory disorder.

As was described in Chapter 2, there are three basic mechanisms of memory. The first is encoding, namely, laying down new memories in the brain. The mechanisms of concentration and focusing attention are essential to insuring that encoding is done properly. The second is storage, the storage of memories in the memory banks of the brain. The third is retrieval, the retrieval of memories from the memory bank for our use.

Panic and depression interfere with the encoding of new memories. They interfere with concentration and focusing of attention. If new memories are not properly encoded, they will not be stored properly in the memory bank. Finally, the retrieval of deficient memories from the widespread memory bank is also going to be seriously impaired.

Unfortunately, bad conditioned reflexes, particularly those that are associated with strong emotions like fear and anger, are easily remembered and are very easy to retrieve. In a paradoxical way, these bad memories, which are so easily accessible to us even when we don't want them, have a particularly noxious effect on the laying down of new memories, good memories that we need and that may be vital to us.

To further compound the problem, the bad conditioned reflexes and the memories that go along with them may impair our memory process to such a great extent that we believe we are developing Alzheimer's disease. Unfortunately, the panic and depression that sets in with this false belief impairs our memory process even more.

Efforts on our part to block out the bad memories with alcohol, marijuana, cocaine, or other street drugs may make the memory loss even worse because all of these drugs have various poisonous effects on brain function, and ultimately memory abilities will suffer. Even some prescription drugs, particularly those that are used to relieve anxiety, may depress brain function and memory. This doesn't mean that all medicines used to treat depression and anxiety are bad or inappropriate. However, it is very important to reach an accurate diagnosis of what the trouble is and use treatments that are least likely to be harmful to the brain.

Once bad conditioned reflexes and their associated memories are set up, it can be very difficult to remove them. But there are techniques for diminishing their importance and procedures for overcoming their bad effects, as we saw with Shane and Jennifer.

Bad memories and their bad conditioned reflexes are among the most frequent causes of memory dysfunction. Because of the many different kinds of conditioned reflexes that develop in human beings, it is not possible to outline all the different therapeutic approaches that can be used to correct this kind of dysfunction. However, most often the bad conditioned reflexes and the bad memories that go with them are triggered by feelings of loss of control. The elements of the therapeutic approach to problems of this sort do have some general themes.

First, it is critical to take a good history, with an emphasis on identifying issues related to a loss of control. Second, a general physical examination should be carried out. Third, a neurological examination should be done, which should include a mental status examination.

Generally, a mental status examination consists of the following kinds of investigations: orientation as to time, place, and person; the repetition of test phrases; the carrying out of crossover commands; the understanding of written and spoken speech; the performance of mental arithmetic; the changing of sets; the testing of remote memory; the testing of recent memory; and the ability to remember four unrelated words, after an interval of four minutes, during which time the subject is performing other aspects of the mental status exam.

If the mental status examination shows no evidence of a memory problem, and yet the subject still complains of this, a more detailed neuropsychological test should be given. If, on the other hand, the mental status examination shows only the dysfunction of recent memory, the program described in this chapter should be initiated. That is, a program of simple and finally complex memory exercises should be begun. Simultaneously, a program of cortical brain relaxation, as described in this chapter, should be started.

Finally, it is my recommendation that the program of memory exercise and cortical brain relaxation should be done as a preventive measure in people who do not have symptoms of memory loss. Just as people without heart disease run to keep their hearts in shape or lift weights to keep their muscles strong, people should exercise their memory abilities and their cortical relaxation conditioned reflex to keep their brains working at top efficiency. Good conditioned reflexes are always useful. The more of them that we develop, the better. And good conditioned reflexes that reinforce our memory abilities are especially important for our continued mental health.

5

Memory Loss and Aging

HAVE YOU NOTICED that as you've gotten older you've become more set in your ways? Well, it's hardly surprising then that your father and mother, or grandparents if they're still alive, have the same problem. If they had poor memories when they were young, their memories may have become terrible in their advanced years. But is this problem just a function of getting older, or is it a medical condition for which they should be receiving treatment? Do their memory problems indicate a brain abnormality? And, more important, are their problems treatable and reversible?

Where Does It Begin?

Physicians working at a research center in St. Louis, Missouri, recently completed a study of eighty-two elderly volunteers to determine whether normal, healthy people deteriorate as they grow older. The study was carried out in such a fashion that some of the patients were studied for up to fifteen years and six months. They were evaluated by a clinical dementia rating scale, which is a psychometric test that shows whether or not a person has signs of dementia. The rating scale is not conclusive, that is, it won't prove whether or not someone has dementia, but over a long period of time it can accurately measure significant changes in brain function. In the St. Louis study the volunteers were given ninety-minute batteries of psychometric tests on a repeated basis.

Some interesting results were reported. The participants with poorer performance on psychometric testing (defined as Minimal Cognitive Impairment [MCI]) at the time of enrollment were at a higher risk for intellectual decline subsequently. As years went by, when a subtle intellectual decline was detected clinically, an abrupt deterioration in the performance on independently administered psychometric tests was seen.

The main finding of the study was that intellectually healthy elderly people maintained stable intellectual performance, as measured over a period of years by both careful clinical evaluation and repeated psychometric testing. Their stability was maintained unless or until they developed a dementing illness, at which time a sharp decline in performance was observed. This is clearly good news, as it's an indication that dementia is not a part of normal aging.

Other kinds of tests generally support this view. A review of memory performance in aging, done by psychologists at Pomona College in Claremont, California, showed a consistent pattern of spared and impaired memory abilities in normal old age. Relatively preserved as people get older is memory performance involving highly practiced skills and familiar information, which includes factual, semantic, and autobiographical information. Relatively impaired in old age is memory performance that requires the formation of new connections, for example, the recall of recent autobiographical experiences, new facts, or the source of newly acquired facts. This pattern of impaired new learning versus preserved old learning cuts across distinctions between semantic memory, episodic memory, and other kinds of memory.

What these findings all indicate is that you have to keep using your memory, or it will rapidly deteriorate. So, it's clear from psychological research that there are both theoretical and

empirical reasons for emphasizing practice and familiariza-
tion skills as a strategy for maintaining and improving intellectual functions in old age.

Age seems to affect certain kinds of memory more than
others. For example, while elderly subjects did worse than
younger subjects in recognizing odors, when tested by naming
an odor and giving a short description, they were the equal of
the younger test subjects in terms of associating a memory of a
life episode with each odor. In regard to remembering visual
stimuli, older subjects were able to demonstrate short-term retention of visual stimuli across a time line of one to four seconds just as well as younger subjects. In fact, those visual
abilities that were dependent upon visual cortex and not retinal factors remained relatively unchanged despite age-related
changes in the eyeball. Visual memory functions that were dependent upon working and long-term memory abilities, on
the other hand, showed a significant age-associated decline
during adulthood.

For the past several years, scientists have been looking
for an easy way to diagnose Alzheimer's disease, and some
promising new research indicates that there may be a substance found only in the blood of Alzheimer's victims. The
substance is called apolipoprotein-E genotype with epsilon
four allele. The results of an Italian study showed that, for reasons that are not clear, more women with Alzheimer's disease
had the epsilon four allele than did men. There was also a statistically significant increase in epsilon four frequency in patients with the late onset of Alzheimer's disease as compared
to the rest of the groups. And there was some increased frequency of epsilon four in both probable and possible late-
onset Alzheimer's disease. However, there was no similar
trend in vascular dementia, or in age-associated memory impairment. All of this indicates that it is still extremely difficult
to make an exact diagnosis of Alzheimer's, although there are

positive indications that a simple blood test may eventually be possible.

Today, unfortunately, the most conclusive evidence of Alzheimer's is still the clinical pathology work done for a post-mortem examination. Recently a pathological study was carried out in St. Louis, Missouri, that demonstrated the relation of histological markers to dementia severity, age, sex, and the apolipoprotein-E genotype. This was done in patients who were followed clinically until their deaths. Post-mortem examinations were done on all the patients, and a detailed study of the patients' brains was carried out.

The researchers found a striking relationship between neurofibrillary tangles in the brain and advanced Alzheimer's disease. These tangles, seen in post-mortem, were the most common pathology associated with Alzheimer's. Advanced age at death was associated with somewhat less severe dementia and fewer pathological changes. Despite a substantial effect of apolipoprotein-E epsilon four as a risk factor for Alzheimer's disease, on decreasing the age of onset for Alzheimer's disease and increasing the amount of the protein deposit amyloid, resulting from tissue degeneration, in the brain, the effect of epsilon four on the neuropathological changes of the brain was variable and complex. This is currently a very interesting area for Alzheimer's research.

There are some clinicians who feel that such changes, which differentiate Alzheimer's disease from normal aging, are present in the Alzheimer's patients years before clinical symptoms appear. I am not convinced, however, that all the evidence is in. When my grandfather had severe memory loss in his eighties resulting from Alzheimer's disease, I was tempted to look back at the symptoms of personality change that had occurred ten to fifteen years before the disease was diagnosed. Did those symptoms indicate the beginning of Alzheimer's? The more I thought about it, the more I was sure that they probably did not. The changes he went through were likely related to his grief for the death of his wife of over forty years more than anything else.

Memory loss in an elderly person may begin in such a subtle or gradual fashion that the resulting personality change or disability is difficult to differentiate from the more usual day-to-day fluctuations in performance. It can manifest itself in such things as missing meals, with weight loss or malnutrition, or a change in dressing habits, neatness, cleanliness, or hygiene. Are these reasons to seek medical help, considering that the elderly person is likely to react angrily to the suggestion that he or she should see a doctor about any of these problems?

In younger people, memory loss may appear suddenly, especially after a head injury or a bout of alcohol or drug abuse. Sometimes it occurs after someone is put on medication for sleeplessness or anxiety, which results from depression. Should anyone with these problems seek medical attention?

The decision about whether someone has a genuine memory deficiency is not an easy one to make. Even doctors have memory problems, so don't be discouraged if this gray area between brain abnormalities and social or psychological influences seems confusing and imprecise. It is. There are, however, some things we can do to help.

First, we can sort out the memory complaints that do not usually indicate serious brain difficulties and are unlikely to require examination by a physician. It is, of course, not uncommon or unusual for anyone to have trouble remembering things from time to time. If you have any of the following problems, in the absence of any other symptoms, you most likely do not need to consult a doctor:

- forgetting names
- misplacing keys, glasses, or other small items

- not being able to find your car in a parking lot
- not being able to remember items to shop for at the store
- not being able to recognize someone in an unfamiliar setting

What follows is a list of memory problems and the changes that occur in function and personality. These symptoms do require medical investigation:

- getting lost while driving a familiar route
- completely forgetting important appointments
- telling the same stories over and over to the same people during a short space of time (i.e., no short-term recall)
- having periods of confusion over what time it is or where one is
- being unable to manage a checkbook or take care of simple finances
- experiencing a sudden or gradual change in personality
- having difficulty with language (e.g., naming objects)
- experiencing a sudden change in artistic or musical ability
- undergoing a loss of memory which is disabling to the point that work is impossible or one's daily activity level is upset

To answer questions about the significance of memory loss, whether in the young or the old, more fully, you or a friend or relative can carry out some preliminary testing for yourself (or on each other). The following self-help test of mental status will help you determine if an examination by a neurologist is necessary. The steps are simple on paper, but they may be difficult to carry out if the person you suspect may have a memory problem is much older than you are; if you are both unsure of your motives and become defensive or uncooperative; or if either of you is too confused to follow the instructions or is humiliated by the testing process.

If you can't complete all of the test, respond to as many of the entries as you can. Sometimes subjects' responses, even when they aren't right, can give others an intuitive feeling about the significance of their memory difficulties.

Here is the sample test:

1. Give your friend or relative three words to remember — for example, table, lamp, flower — and ask that they be repeated after five minutes of doing other mental tasks.
2. See whether your friend knows what the date is and where exactly you both are.
3. Have the person repeat the phrase "No ifs, ands, or buts."
4. Have the person name and identify common objects — for example, a ring, a pencil, glasses, and the like.
5. Ask the person to draw the face of a clock and put the numbers in the proper positions.
6. Have the person subtract sixteen from one hundred and multiply thirteen by twelve.
7. Ask the person to interpret the proverb "A stitch in time saves nine."
8. Have your friend name the current president of the United States and the preceding six presidents in reverse order.
9. Have him or her read a paragraph from a book, magazine, or newspaper and explain what the passage means.
10. Ask the person to name the states that border your state.

You might wonder why this kind of formal testing is necessary if you already suspect that the person you're worried about has a problem. Since you've observed your friend's muddled thinking and memory problems at close range, isn't that enough? The answer is that your subjective impressions, or even the impressions of a trained professional, such as a doctor, may turn out to be wrong. Testing done in the manner described above — that is, formal testing of mental status — gives some objective basis for a decision about what's wrong.

If your friend or relative "passes" this simple test, the person probably doesn't need to see a neurologist, despite complaints about poor memory. But if your friend cannot respond accurately to all the questions, it may be that his or her degree of memory loss and personality change is significant. It is important to carry out neurological testing in anyone who has suffered genuine memory loss and personality change, whatever the person's age — but more especially in those who are elderly. My own clinical investigations of elderly people with personality change and beginning memory loss, however, often reveal no evidence of Alzheimer's disease but rather clinical problems that are the result of some other cause — one that is frequently treatable.

Danny, seventy-nine, was referred by one of my physician acquaintances to the center I co-founded for the treatment of memory impairment. His daughter was very worried about his living alone because when she visited him he often seemed bewildered. Danny would, for example, open the cellar door of his house rather than the closet door to put his coat away. He also became confused whenever he drove to the next state to visit his daughter.

He was a retired real estate broker and scoutmaster who had no demands on his time. And because he lived alone he was careless about preparing meals and sometimes didn't eat much for two or three days at a time.

From his medical history, I had anticipated that he might be a candidate for enrollment in a therapeutic trial of an anti-Alzheimer's drug. But even minimal testing showed that his mental status was much too good for him to be classified as being in the beginning stages of Alzheimer's. In fact, Danny was suffering from depression.

The steps we at the center took with him are the same that

would be taken with any elderly person who is failing to thrive, especially one recently widowed or bereaved. First, we got him a dog. Having to care for an animal imposed a routine on Danny's life because the dog had to be fed and walked regularly, and he was a constant companion. Next we insisted that Danny take up being a scoutmaster again. He also reestablished social ties through his church, where he went to at least two functions a week which offered not only nourishing food but companionship. And we got him to start a mild exercise routine, with activities he could easily do on a daily basis. Finally, we contacted his physician, who reviewed the dosages of his medications — particularly the drugs he was taking for hypertension — and gave him a daily menu to help maintain his nutrition.

Danny's prescription to regain mental health should be used by anyone who is beginning to drop out or lose motivation. This is especially true if the person performs well on a mental status test but continues to have memory and other mental symptoms. To generalize the advice I gave to Danny, I recommend the following to anyone in his position:

- Establish a routine. Having a pet, such as a dog, is a good way to do this.
- Reestablish social ties through a church or voluntary organization.
- Make sure meals are nutritious; join Meals on Wheels or some other program if food preparation is a problem.
- Consult your doctor about medications and diet.
- Start a mild exercise program (e.g., brisk walking) if possible.

The above suggestions in no way substitute for medical, psychiatric, or neurological management when it is needed.

However, they are an important supplement to any program to maintain well-being for persons with memory symptoms but no neurological or medical disease.

I tell my patients never to give up hope, even if they are given a diagnosis of Alzheimer's disease, because some treatable conditions, like the pseudodementia of depression, can mimic Alzheimer's closely. In the early stages at least, it is almost impossible to tell them apart. If you have any doubt about what is wrong, get a second opinion from a neurologist and follow the clinical steps listed later in this chapter.

Competence

No sight is more pathetic than watching relatives squabble over the estate of a victim of memory loss in probate court, attempting to declare him or her incompetent. Psychiatrists hired by one side will say one thing, and psychiatrists on the other side precisely the opposite. The plain truth of the matter is that a diagnosis of Alzheimer's is not equivalent to mental incompetence. And Alzheimer's victims can continue, with assistance, to manage many of their affairs until they have lost significant portions of their vital memories. Finding out whether someone is or isn't competent is by no means a clear-cut process.

What would you do if you or a family member suffered memory loss? In order to determine what the appropriate course of action should be, a number of specific questions need to be asked and answered. For example, do you or anyone in your family have a loss of vital memory? That is, does the person not just forget someone's name or the items on a shopping list, but rather has he or she undergone a loss of orientation? Is the person aware of what happened yesterday? What he or she has to do today? What the prospects for tomorrow are?

If someone in your family has this kind of problem, he or

she needs immediate help. But don't assume that the clinical situation is hopeless or that the chances for recovery are slight, because they're not. Several different disorders can cause vital-memory problems, and many of them are easily treatable: such entities as clinical depression, brain poisoning with alcohol or street drugs (including amphetamines, cocaine, barbiturates, marijuana, Angel Dust, and a variety of drugs prescribed by physicians), nutritional problems like malnutrition and dehydration, and a variety of medical and even neurological disorders. Most of these medical conditions can produce some loss of vital memory, but the loss varies depending on the severity of the problem.

Before I discuss some of these problems in detail, let me also point out that there can sometimes be two or more causes for lapses in vital memory, all of which contribute to a loss of intellectual function. For example, a person who has poisoned his or her brain with alcohol may also suffer from a vitamin B-1 deficiency, have had a head injury, and be subject to epileptic seizures. Each of these problems can impair or reduce vital memory.

Sadly, too, many doctors are trained to look only for the chief cause of a problem, and they fail to dig deeper to discover contributing factors. Your best defense against an incomplete diagnosis is to insist on thorough medical testing and analysis. The following paragraphs explain what you need to know and what you should expect from a competent diagnostician.

Doctors Who Investigate Memory Lapses

Doctors come with a variety of labels, but these labels don't tell you much about a physician's competence or diligence. A family physician, or generalist, may be more effective and persistent in diagnostic efforts than a high-powered specialist who looks too narrowly at one symptom and misses an underlying cause or a treatable problem. Many family physicians have special training in internal medicine and geriatrics, and some, like the family physicians at the University of Oklahoma Medical School branch in Tulsa, take a special interest in the diagnosis and treatment of reversible causes of memory loss and dementia.

Geriatricians usually have a background in internal medicine and have been examined in all areas of internal medicine, particularly those dealing with heart and lung disease, liver disease, kidney disease, and rheumatology. Some are very interested in the nervous system and good at the differential diagnosis and treatment of memory loss and dementing illness. Others prefer to focus on diseases of the heart, lungs, or joints. These doctors should refer patients suspected of having dementing illness to a specialist in that area.

Most physicians trained in neurology are well equipped to investigate the causes of memory loss and dementing illness and to carry out appropriate treatment. But some board-certified neurologists are criticized because their clinical interests are so narrow that they may miss a potentially treatable cause of dementing illness. Some neurologists, for example, specialize in muscle diseases and their treatment, and they're not interested in the degenerative diseases of the brain. If a physician doesn't try to find every possible cause of memory loss in making a neurological evaluation, he or she is not the doctor for you. You will need another neurologist.

Psychiatrists come in all shapes and sizes. In recent years the new field of geriatric psychiatry has emerged. Psychiatrists in this field are especially expert in treating depression in the elderly and also in psychopharmacology, the art and science of balancing medications to give the most beneficial effects and the fewest side effects. Most geriatric psychiatrists demand a complete evaluation of a patient's medical and neurological state before they will undertake any definitive treatment. But this is not true of all psychiatrists. Some

79

psychiatrists ignore potentially treatable medical problems and correctable neurological ailments, much to the detriment of their patients' well-being.

Psychologists often treat patients with group psychotherapy or various environmental psychotherapies in the nursing home setting. They also carry out various kinds of psychological testing. They are not physicians, however, and they should not begin a treatment program on any patient with dementing illness until the patient has had a complete medical and neurological evaluation.

An Optimal Test of Vital Memory

With these factors in mind, my partner, Tom Sabin, a neurologist, and I began the Center for Memory Impairment and Neurobehavioral Disturbances (CMIND), sold in 1995 and later closed by a hospital chain. The center's chief effort was to examine patients with memory loss and disabling dementia, or other forms of behavioral disturbance, before rather than after they were committed to nursing homes. We have also examined many residents of nursing homes to try to find treatable problems, lessen their symptoms, and make the lives of these patients both more comfortable and more rewarding.

One thing we require for every patient is as complete a medical history as possible, and this is often difficult to get. The histories of patients in nursing homes have often been lost, and significant factors may not come to light during a diagnostic evaluation. Second, we do a number of blood tests to screen for various conditions — anemia, malnutrition, diabetes, thyroid impairment, syphilis, electrolyte imbalance — and get appropriate medical evaluations when these tests disclose some problem.

Next we have the patient psychologically tested for evidence of emotional problems such as severe depression. Finally, we take the blood levels of all medications the patient is on which can cause memory loss or other dementing illness.

If the patient exhibits some evidence of depression, we have him or her seen by a geriatric psychiatrist for evaluation for psychotherapy or other appropriate therapy.

A neurological examination and if necessary a brain wave test (that is, an electroencephalogram) are done on the patient, along with a visualization of the brain itself in a CAT or MRI scan as well as neuropsychological testing, giving a detailed analysis of memory function. Most important, we have a senior member of our staff correlate the findings from all the examinations. In writing an integrated summary report to the referring physician, this doctor lists the pertinent findings from each examination and offers medical recommendations, which may include a drug "holiday," new medications, psychotherapy, a change in the patient's residence or in his or her relationships with, for example, family members. At times a surgical or operative lesion such as hydrocephalus, a brain tumor, or a blood clot (subdural hematoma) is found pressing on the brain and it must then be removed.

I have not discussed all the tests that might need to be done on each patient. For example, some patients may need a spinal tap or lumbar puncture to look at their spinal fluid. Not every patient needs every test. The evaluation still depends on the physician's knowledge and judgment, but we think the CMIND paradigm is appropriate not only for determining whether a patient should be sent to a nursing home, but for assessing the condition of many patients already in such facilities.

National Policy Issues

The present diagnosis and treatment of elderly patients with memory loss is often inadequate, and the medical approach is just part of the answer to a perplexing and difficult problem. Social and economic solutions are also needed, including, for example, intergenerational housing, that is, semidetached housing that would accommodate three generations in a single family. But of course such solutions address a wider problem than memory loss. Nevertheless, memory loss is a salient symptom of the hundreds of thousands of elderly persons who now challenge us to provide better medical and diagnostic treatment centers in the United States.

Needless to say, the more people we can keep out of nursing homes the better. If we can slow down or reverse memory loss, everyone gains. It is important to keep people active and contributing to society, and older individuals, because of the richness of their experience, have much to offer the rest of us. It is doubly necessary that we determine the precise cause of memory loss and dementing illness as quickly as symptoms appear so that appropriate medical steps can be taken. The cost of not doing this, in decreasing the quality of the patient's life as well as increasing the financial burden on all the rest of us, makes any other alternative unthinkable.

Finally, when considering national policy issues and the cost of preventing and reversing memory loss, we have to remember that we are now dealing with more than just an elderly population. The "baby boom" generation has reached the age where memory loss is increasingly a reason for medical consultation. People in their fifties frequently have some elderly relatives with the symptoms of progressive memory loss. And whenever the "boomers" forget where they put their glasses or their car keys, they immediately think that the worst is happening to them — that they're getting Alzheimer's disease.

The causes of their memory loss may not be significant, but the very fact that they can't remember as quickly or as accurately as they did before puts them at a disadvantage in our intensely competitive society. Fortunately, most are not shy about asking for professional help in keeping their memory functions intact.

Nevertheless, while the cost of this medical assistance is small for each individual, there are so many people of this age in our population that the total cost could become very substantial. Furthermore, if the beginning symptoms of memory loss are neglected, sufferers may become depressed and suffer more severe memory loss. The eventual cost of treatment will be substantially greater than if the symptoms are treated when they first occur. Therefore, it is important for everyone with symptoms of memory impairment to get at least an early memory screening test to detect any memory problems that will not just disappear with the passage of time — problems that will require a more accurate diagnosis and the initiation of effective treatments. The costs of the memory screening tests are minimal, especially compared to the benefits from getting an early and accurate diagnosis of potentially major future problems.

Vital Memory Points to Remember

Which memory symptoms are probably not significant?

It is not uncommon or unusual for anyone to have trouble remembering things from time to time. If you have any of the following problems, in the absence of any other symptoms, you most likely do not need to consult a doctor:

- forgetting names
- misplacing keys, glasses, or other small items
- not being able to find your car in a parking lot
- not being able to remember items to shop for at the store
- not being able to recognize someone in an unfamiliar setting

Which memory symptoms do require medical investigation?

If you have any of the following symptoms you should have a medical professional check you out:

- getting lost while driving a familiar route
- completely forgetting important appointments
- telling the same stories over and over to the same people during a short space of time (i.e., no short-term recall)
- having periods of confusion over what time it is or where you are
- being unable to manage a checkbook or take care of simple finances
- experiencing a sudden or gradual change in personality
- having difficulty with language (e.g., naming objects)
- experiencing a sudden change in artistic or musical ability
- undergoing a loss of memory which is disabling to the point that work is impossible or your daily activity level is upset

What should you do if your symptoms require medical investigation?

1. Ask your doctor to refer you to a neurologist. If you don't have a doctor, call your local medical society and ask for a referral to a neurologist specializing in problems of memory loss and dementing illness.
2. When you see the neurologist, make certain that a full mental status examination, *including memory testing*, is done. If the results are not completely normal, the neurologist will refer you to a neuropsychologist for detailed memory testing.
3. If the results of your memory test aren't normal, you will also need a complete physical examination, including blood and urine tests to determine levels of the medications you are on. Furthermore, you will need a complete neurological examination in which a detailed history of your problem, together with an accurate medical history, is taken.

4. If these tests are not completely normal, you should have a CAT or MRI scan of the brain as well as an electroencephalogram and possibly a lumbar puncture. Detailed neuropsychological tests, if not already done, should complete this evaluation.

What should you do if problems arise?

1. If your physician or neurologist is unwilling to have these tests done, you must find a physician who will do them.
2. If the results of these tests are normal and you still have a pattern of memory loss, you should consult a geriatric psychiatrist to establish whether depression is present and, if so, how it should be treated.
3. If your doctor does not sit down with you to review all the medications you are taking and how they might be contributing to your problem, you must find a doctor who will.
4. If after all the above steps are carried out you have symptoms of memory loss and still were not given a diagnosis, you should repeat the evaluation in three to six months.
5. A complete and thorough evaluation should identify the cause of any memory loss. Then, either the loss can be reversed by appropriate treatment or further progression of memory loss can be prevented.
6. Even if a progressive disease like Alzheimer's is found, a number of measures can be taken to prolong the useful life of an Alzheimer's patient, including:
   - diagnosing and treating other causes of dementia which make the symptoms of Alzheimer's worse
   - helping the patient establish and keep a routine around times and places
   - making orienting aids such as large calendars and clocks available
   - allowing the Alzheimer's patient as much freedom as

possible compatible with safety (e.g., doors to the outside should be locked, but doors to and from the bathroom or bedroom should stay open)

7. One should always allow Alzheimer's patients to remain as productive as possible for as long as they can function effectively. For example, one Alzheimer's patient constantly got lost coming back from the bathroom but could still make sound decisions about investments. Another patient could hardly talk yet managed to plant a beautiful flower garden. Remember that a person's having a diagnosis of Alzheimer's does not mean that he or she is necessarily incompetent, by either a clinical or a legal definition. The individual's competence depends on the state and extent of brain disease.

6

Depression: A Common Cause of Reversible Vital Memory Loss and Intellectual Deterioration

YOU MAY HAVE a poor or failing memory that interferes not only with achievement of your hopes and aspirations but also with your everyday performance. But do you know what is causing your memory difficulty? Although a precise diagnosis often depends on appropriate medical and psychological testing, you can begin to get some idea of the cause by looking at the kind of memory problem you have as well as at some of the other problems in your life which have coincided with your memory loss.

Do you find that you have difficulty learning new things? Do you have difficulty concentrating? Are you easily distracted so that the focus of your attention wavers? In other words, do you have a short attention span? Do you feel that you try to force your mental processes to function efficiently, only to find yourself bogged down like a prize fighter trying to throw a punch under water? Do you feel anxious or have difficulty sleeping? Do you wake up very early in the morning, well before you want to? Do you find yourself worried or upset? Do things look hopeless, as though there is no end to your troubles and you will never be able to work your way out of difficulty? If you are having memory difficulties along with these kinds of symptoms, it is likely that your problem is caused in large part by depression.

An example of this kind of problem was presented by Thelma, a sixty-three-year-old widow, who told me, "Doctor, I can't remember anything. It's a good thing I live right next to the grocery store because I have to go back three or four times a day just to remember the things I was supposed to shop for. I finally started making a list, but then I forgot it and had to go back home to get it."

When I took Thelma's history, it turned out that her problems with memory had started about four weeks before she saw me. This was a tip-off that something that had happened recently changed her level of functioning. More important, no unusual medical problem had arisen to produce this sudden change in her level of competence. So I began to probe her life situation: did she have problems with her children? The answer was no. Thelma assured me that she didn't smoke or drink and had never taken drugs. What about her finances? Well, she lived on a widow's pension and had been just able to get by until about a month before. What happened at that time? She had gotten her property tax bill on her tiny little bungalow; her taxes had gone up dramatically and tipped her precarious money situation toward bankruptcy. She told me, "Doctor, my husband Sam and I worked all our lives to save a little something, and now it's all gone. Now the town is going to take away my house."

My treatment of Thelma was not medical but rather social and political. I got in touch with one of the senior town officials, who told me he would do everything he could to help her. The very fact that something could be done, and was being done, elevated her spirits and improved her level of memory functioning. Thelma had a reversible kind of memory loss, probably the most common and the most easily misdiagnosed one — that is, memory loss associated with depression. There are, in fact, several forms of depression, and all produce some loss of memory and reduction of previous intellectual capacities. But all forms of depression don't act equally to reduce vital memory.

Doctors often classify depression by its severity. No matter what the cause, the most severe forms produce a profound loss of vital memory. The least severe, on the other hand, do not impair vital memory, but other forms of memory may be affected. It shouldn't be surprising that this is the case. Almost all of us know how a feeling of depression can impair our day-to-day functioning. Our efficiency is reduced, we don't pay attention to what people say to us, our personal finances may fall into disarray, paying bills for things like taxes and insurance may not get done, and we stop our routine and may not even get to work.

There are other classifications of depression. Cases related to life adjustment problems are psychological in origin. Doctors frequently observe grief reactions, for example, when patients lose spouses, parents, or children, or others who are close to them. Some doctors witness "burnout" syndrome when depressed patients become discouraged with the jobs they're in and don't see any future, or when they are severely stressed by their jobs and find no way of achieving success, looking forward only to increasing demands and unpleasant responsibilities. Such stress-induced depression can often be treated by various forms of psychotherapy or environmental change (for example, changing a job) Often it is self-limited.

Depression in the elderly related to life adjustment problems can be very disabling because many elderly persons lack the resources and the recuperative powers of the young, and moreover their symptoms can mimic dementia and thus be misdiagnosed. In the early stages of the disorder, increased support from relatives and friends may stop the downward slide before the patient goes into deep depression, requiring antidepressants and professional psychotherapy to remedy.

Other kinds of depression seem to be related not to a stressful environment but rather to some abnormality in brain chemistry or neurotransmitter function — in other words, to some problem in the brain itself. Sometimes patients who have this kind of depression find that other members of their families — parents, grandparents, brothers, sisters, cousins — have the same complaints. At times the depression is accompanied by severe mood swings; that is, periods of elation and manic activity, which are followed by depression. Here too there may be a family history of this disorder, which, strangely enough, is often associated with high intelligence and a record of achievement. Some forms of depression, finally, seem to be related to menopause, which may also trigger neurochemical changes in the brain.

All of these brain-related forms of depression can produce some loss of vital memory, but the important point to remember is that they are treatable, and the lives and memories of patients suffering from these symptoms can be greatly improved. The following sections describe the more typical clinical pictures of depression and vital memory loss, the kind of problem that brings people to hospitals and, if unrecognized and untreated, sends them to nursing homes.

Clinical Depression and Memory Loss

When most of us think of a person who is depressed, we get a mental image of someone who is tearful, slowed down, almost apathetic, not moving much, possibly sitting or lying down, just staring blankly off into space. Although some severely depressed people are like that, many of the ten million persons in the United States who have suffered from clinical depression sometime during their lives behave somewhat differently. They may feel hopeless and have a sense that things are closing in on them. Usually they seem agitated. Sleep disturbances are quite common, and often they wake up early in the morning and can't get back to sleep.

When such persons come to see a doctor they appear to be more anxious than depressed, and it is not uncommon for the doctor to prescribe a tranquilizer and a sleeping pill. Unfortunately, these medications not only don't bring the patient out of the depressed state but may make it much worse.

Billy, a fifty-three-year-old machinist, was one of my patients who had this happen to him. Over a number of years, Billy became more and more concerned about losing his memory. He thought he was following in the steps of his father, who had memory lapses before the age of sixty and who finally suffered profound dementia leading to premature death. Billy had always been an independent sort of person, steady and hard-working, but his life had been beset by troubles. His first wife died of cancer, leaving him with a ten-year-old daughter to raise, and his second marriage was unhappy and finally ended in divorce a month before he came to talk with me.

When I saw him the first thing I noticed was that Billy had trouble relaxing. Everything was in motion — his hands, feet, arms, and torso; he looked like a four-year-old who couldn't sit still. He was playing with his glasses, and he seemed overly sensitive to any change in my mood or manner when I spoke to him. Even though his chief complaint was his memory loss, he also told me that he had trouble sleeping at night and that he woke up at five-thirty in the morning and couldn't get back to sleep. He looked bleary-eyed, and he said his work was deteriorating. On some days he couldn't go to work at all. Finally he admitted that he had been trying to treat his memory problem with increasing amounts of alcohol. (Incidentally, it is extremely common for depressed patients to medicate themselves with alcohol, cocaine, amphetamines, or other street drugs. The initial drug- or alcohol-induced euphoria is often followed by deeper depression, which is even more resistant to subsequent doses of drugs or alcohol.) Of course, the alcohol didn't work; it just made him more depressed as well as alcohol-dependent.

The reason for Billy's depression was fairly obvious from his history. The dissolution of his stormy marriage, his only daughter's living with a semi-alcoholic man, financial troubles, and threatened layoffs at work all contributed to a very real environmental stress–related depression. On top of this, he began to perceive his own mortality as he approached sixty, the age at which his father's mental powers had begun to decline.

Seeing how agitated he was, it would have been the easiest thing in the world to give him some sleeping pills, or Valium, or Ativan. But what he really needed was problem resolution — someone to talk to his boss to find out what his chances for continued employment were (they turned out to be good), and family counseling sessions for him and his daughter. It helped that she was quite sensitive to her father's problems, and even though her living arrangements didn't change to suit him completely, the sessions at least allowed Billy and his daughter to achieve a more comfortable relationship.

In this case, the patient's problems could be resolved by his talking things out with someone skilled in psychotherapy. When his troubles were approached in this way, Billy's memory complaints disappeared and his sleep patterns returned to normal. Moreover, he became much less anxious and fearful than he had been. His anxiety level decreased immediately after his problem was explained, and his first good night's sleep followed shortly thereafter. The noticeable improvement in his memory took almost two weeks, and it came as a very pleasant surprise to him.

Memory Defects in Depression

We all have life adjustment problems, of course, and from time to time each of us is susceptible to mild depression. What we have to remember is that if we suddenly become forgetful, or if memory loss becomes a major concern to us, we should first try to discover if the real underlying problem is depression.

Depression affects the memory process in several different ways. Most important, it is often associated with hyperdistractibility; we just have too much on our minds. A depressed individual, even one with mild depression, is less able to focus attention and concentrate. Environmental impulses are thus much less likely to be formed into memory engrams in the brain, and even if engrams are formed, because information processing has been somewhat interfered with, they are defective. The neuropsychologist might call these defective engrams shallow memory traces. Because they are less permanent, the rate of forgetting is increased. In other words, their storage in the memory bank in any useful form is less likely.

Another defect in the memory mechanism which is common in depressed patients is that they are slow to retrieve specific memories. This can be true even though they often don't show any loss of memory at a more generalized level. Retrieving and reconstituting memories from their memory banks is a chore, although eventually they are able to dredge up the information they're searching for.

Depression, then, produces several defects in memory processing. Because of hyperdistractibility and lack of concentration it interferes with acquisition of new memories. It also interferes with retrieval from the memory bank and reconstitution, so that recall also becomes defective.

Some psychologists claim that memory impairment is not present in mild cases of depression, but this is certainly not my experience. For example, the case history of a long-time family friend, Clarence, demonstrates that mild and easily remedied depression can produce annoying changes in memory abilities.

I had known Clarence since the time both our families lived in the same city. He was an extremely bright and capable electrical engineer and certainly one of the nicest people I have ever known. After he left the air force he went to work for a Defense Department contractor, and about two years ago he retired to live in California.

He had always prided himself on his superior memory, but Clarence called me recently to say he was having great difficulty remembering the names of persons whose faces he was familiar with. He added, ominously, that the problem was getting worse.

I went over a number of possible factors — his daily activities, his diet, his challenges — and found one particular area that was disturbing him. His wife of many years, who was four or five years younger than he, also prided herself on her ability to remember names. They were walking together on a beach one day when they encountered an old acquaintance whose name Clarence could not remember. His wife, however, came up with the name immediately. Clarence gradually came to the conclusion that he was losing his memory when this same sequence was repeated several times over. This in turn precipitated a reactive depression that made his memory problem much worse.

I told Clarence it wasn't unusual for people as they grow older to have some difficulty recalling names, and that this was true even of persons with superior memories. Furthermore, I told him he sounded depressed, and he admitted it. He finally realized that the cause of his depression was that his wife seemed to have an easier time remembering names than he, which meant to him that he was failing. With this recognition and some dietary changes — the addition of B vitamins and lecithin in concentrated form — I told him to try again and see if things didn't improve.

Three or four weeks later I got a long distance telephone call from Clarence, who was bubbling over with enthusiasm. He said that he and his wife had been walking in a shopping center when they encountered a couple they hadn't seen in years. His wife couldn't come up with the couple's names, but the names appeared in Clarence's mind like magic. While I was pleased that his depression had lifted and his memory abilities returned, I advised him to learn from his experience and not to put so much pressure on himself to remember names, especially in competition with his wife.

Severe Depression

More severe cases of depression produce more intense difficulties with memory. However, it is hard to correlate the degree of memory loss with the degree of depression exactly, partly because of the inexact criteria for gauging the intensity of the depressed state. Many psychologists and even psychiatrists feel that the suicidal patient suffers the most intense of the forms of depression. Here again, my experience says otherwise. There is a deeper depression that leaves the patient so apathetic that any meaningful behavior, including a suicide attempt, is almost impossible.

The most severely depressed patient is the one who has psychomotor retardation — an inability to plan for the future or even to move. Such patients will often lie in an almost mute state, unable to feed themselves or to wipe away the tears that well up in their eyes. They may have urinary retention, an inability to empty their bladders. They have a genuine loss of vital memory; testing patients in this state shows that almost all memory processing and intellectual abilities have been impeded. Because of their psychomotor retardation, it is difficult for them to carry out any complex behavior — including an attempt to commit suicide.

When treatment begins, whether it consists of drugs, electroshock treatment, or even surgery, and patients get better — their mood improves, they're able to feed themselves and take care of many of their own needs — at this point in the clinical course the danger of suicide becomes greater. Psychologists, psychiatrists, or other physicians managing these clinical cases must be aware of the potential for this devastating action and take appropriate preventive measures.

Ellen was such a patient. She had been treated by a Harvard psychiatrist for over twenty-five years for recurrent and severe depression. She repeatedly tried psychotherapy and group therapy and had successively taken the whole gamut of antidepressant medications known to physicians at the time. When none of these worked her psychiatrist, who was very conservative, reluctantly called in another specialist to administer electroshock treatments. These produced some transient memory loss, but also a temporary improvement in her depression.

Even with a full complement of medications, Ellen still required four more courses of electroshock treatments during the next ten years to reverse her steadily worsening depression. Because she was deteriorating and her psychiatrist didn't know what else to do, he called on me to operate on the limbic portion of her brain to try to alleviate her depression. When I first saw her she was lying in her bed staring at the ceiling, unable to wipe the tears from her cheeks, unable to urinate, unable to feed herself, unable to drink water, even when a straw was held to her lips.

I performed an operation in which a tiny electrode was inserted into a central area of her brain called the anterior nucleus of the thalamus. There were only two points out of thirty-six electrodes which, when stimulated, produced an exacerbation of anxiety and depression, and these points were destroyed by a tiny heat lesion generated by radio-frequency current.

After surgery, Ellen had a profound loss of recent memory, which lasted for six to eight weeks. When the memory loss began to disappear, however, it was obvious that her depression had substantially lifted. She was able to talk rationally with her psychiatrist, who was enthusiastic about her ability to take care of herself and plan for the future. Clinically she got better and better.

The day came when Ellen was allowed to shop by herself in a downtown department store. In the basement rest room of Filene's she took some poison she had carefully secreted in her handbag and committed suicide.

The effects of surgery had at first been encouraging. Ellen's mood and memory were greatly improved, and her psychomotor retardation was reversed — just the results we wanted from the operation. But surgical treatment contributed only a part, indeed a minor part, to Ellen's therapy. Unfortunately, Ellen's psychiatrist was deceived by the apparent clinical change in his patient. He did not realize that in spite of her remarkable improvement in mood she was still dangerously suicidal. This paradoxical therapeutic effect can be seen with medical as well as surgical therapies of depression. You should bring this fact to the attention of any physician treating a relative or friend of yours for depression. It could save a life. Just remember that an initial improvement in the mood of a severely depressed patient does not necessarily remove the danger of suicide.

Severe Depression in the Elderly

The loss of memory and other intellectual functions in severe depression can be quite profound. This is particularly true in patients who are over the age of fifty-five. Indeed, they may develop a clinical picture indistinguishable from that of the advanced stages of Alzheimer's disease.

Bridey, an eighty-two-year-old woman, had been in the Rose Manor Nursing Home for six years. She shared a room with a woman who had Alzheimer's disease, and the two behaved and acted very similarly. It was impossible to question her because she wouldn't respond appropriately or even obey simple commands. She would sit all day long, staring at the walls, and because she had developed cataracts in the lenses of both eyes what little visual information might have reached her brain was reduced substantially.

Bridey had also been somewhat hard of hearing in both ears for a number of years, so she could communicate only with the help of a hearing aid. In addition, the sensory monotony of the nursing home worsened her depression. She had the annoying habit of turning the clicker on her hearing aid off whenever anyone came around to visit her. This seemed to be the only purposeful thing she did do because she required assistance with most everything else, including feeding and bathroom functions.

In order to communicate with Bridey, I turned her hearing aid on and unwittingly increased the volume all the way up, producing a high-pitched, piercing sound. She roused from her lethargy and turned the hearing aid off, but in doing so said quite clearly, "Stop that racket. Can't you leave me alone?" This fragment of speech was so unlike any response she had ever exhibited — in other examinations, in her clinical history, and in what was thought to be her clinical state as an end-stage Alzheimer's patient with complete memory loss — that I immediately began various treatments for depression.

Over a period of several weeks the treatments with an antidepressant called Prozac became more and more effective. This drug does not have some of the side effects of other antidepressants, but the therapist has to be very patient in using it because it can take up to a couple of months for the effects of the drug to become clinically apparent.* As Bridey became more talkative and more open to therapy, her geriatric psychiatrist discovered the reasons for her depressed state.

The psychiatrist found that Bridey, like many elderly patients who are forced to live in nursing homes, had wanted to conserve her assets for her children. She had therefore transferred those assets to them, leaving herself penniless and a candidate for Medicaid. Sadly, however, once her children had control of her assets they disappeared from her life, leaving her alone, disillusioned, and disappointed in a constricting world in which environmental stimuli were monotonous and uninspiring. She was in a state of partial sensory deprivation compounded by feelings of loss and abandonment by her own children. This was especially disturbing to her because she had been quite close to her children. She had been their sole support when they were growing up, after her alcoholic husband had abandoned the family early in her marriage and was never heard from again.

Bridey's children, a son and a daughter in their forties, each had their own families and interests. The sudden gift of money to them from their mother, who had been a prudent saver and a wise investor, had temporarily diverted them from their family obligations. When they did come to see Bridey they found her in an obviously demented state with very poor memory functions, so they decided there wasn't anything more they could do. But they became much more attentive when they learned the real facts of the case, which helped ensure that their mother would not again slip into a profound depression — what is often called the pseudodementia of depression.

While it certainly helped Bridey, Prozac is not the only

*Prozac may have the paradoxical effect of not averting suicide attempts in a small number of depressed patients whose energy level is improved by the drug.

effective antidepressant. A number of other agents are available, each acting on different aspects of brain chemistry. Some of the more commonly used antidepressants in the elderly population include the tricyclic antidepressants nortriptyline and desipramine. Monoamine oxidase inhibitors are also useful drugs in resistant forms of depression. Lithium, which is usually used for the treatment of manic-depressive disease, is sometimes helpful in preventing a recurrence of depression. However, it has to be used very carefully in elderly patients because of its side effects.

As was shown in the case with Bridey, Prozac, a selective serotonin reuptake inhibitor,* is frequently used to treat depression in the elderly, along with two other selective serotonin reuptake inhibitors, Zoloft and Paxil. Two other drugs with similar but broader actions (serotonin-norepinephrine reuptake inhibitors) are Effexor and Serzone. Another serotonin reuptake inhibitor that has been found to be effective in reversing the depression associated with certain kinds of stroke is the drug trazodone.

One of the more recent medications for the treatment of depression has been the use of a substance that, in the United States, is usually found in health food shops, namely St.-John's-wort, a plant whose scientific name is *Hypericum perforatum*.

St.-John's-wort was recently tested in a randomized, multicenter trial in which the effects of St.-John's-wort were compared to the effects of amitriptyline — a well-recognized antidepressant drug. At the end of the six-week study there was found to be no statistically significant difference between the groups, although there was a tendency for a better response in the amitriptyline group. With regard to tolerability, however, the St.-John's-wort was clearly superior to amitriptyline, particu-

---

*Serotonin is an amine naturally occurring in the brain; it is involved in the transmission of nerve impulses. Drugs that inhibit its uptake in the central nervous system are used to treat depression.

larly in relation to anticholinergic* and central nervous system adverse events. These adverse events were reduced by over 40 percent in the patients taking the St.-John's-wort. The reduced side effects could confer an advantage in improving compliance in depressed patients taking this medication. However, the potential for complications always exists with this medication, as well as all the other drugs used to treat depression.

Some of these agents, however, although they are potent antidepressants, also interfere with the brain's use of acetylcholine, a neurotransmitter associated with the memory process. It is thus possible for an antidepressant to relieve depression and at the same time make memory loss worse. I therefore always urge treating psychiatrists or physicians to be aware of this potential and to adjust dosage and change drugs if it is clinically necessary.

Later I discuss further some of the more widely used antidepressants and their side effects. Here, however, I want to make you aware of what may be an important new treatment in reversing depression and memory loss: a therapy called transcranial electrical brain stimulation (which is *not* the same as electroshock or electroconvulsive therapy). I firmly believe this therapy will prove effective in treating a great number of depressed patients during the next decade and reduce their need for medication. It too will be examined more fully in subsequent chapters.

Stress, Depression, and Memory Loss

At times in life everyone experiences stressful situations: illness, financial difficulties, even physical danger. The initial response to stress is usually heightened awareness and increased vigilance. But if the stress continues for a long period of time, depression sets in. Everything seems to be closing in

---

*"Cholinergic" refers to a drug that can enhance the effects of acetylcholine neurotransmitters in the brain.

on the person, there don't seem to be any options, and a depressed mood almost inevitably results.

As we've seen already, depression is frequently associated with hyperdistractibility, decreased attention span, and decreased concentration, which causes new memories to be improperly encoded in the limbic brain and often makes the retrieval of remote memories from the memory bank slow and inefficient. Another response to severe stress related to depression is that the depressed brain is susceptible to being overwhelmed by shocking events. The combination of depression and severe stress can produce a dramatic loss of memory in what is known as transient global amnesia.

Transient Global Amnesia

Nathan, fifty-two, was a hard-driving businessman with political ambitions. When the incumbent in the district race for state senator dropped out because of ill health, Nathan took the plunge and used his own resources to enter the contest.

Nathan's position of strength, power, and experience in his business dealings gave him the assurance to be successful. In politics, however, his experience was nil. He therefore hired a campaign manager, Phil, who was equally hard-driving and extremely arrogant. Phil took over not only Nathan's campaign but also his life, ordering Nathan's routine and overseeing every facet of his activities. As the relationship became more and more irritating to Nathan, a series of explosive confrontations erupted between Nathan and Phil. Phil was used to such conflicts, but Nathan, who had been accustomed to the more serene atmosphere of commerce, was not. Nathan became very depressed.

Late one morning he decided he'd had enough and called Phil to sever the relationship. A vitriolic shouting match ensued between the two of them, which could be heard all over Nathan's house. His wife noticed he had a confused look on his face when he hung up the telephone, but when she questioned him he said he didn't remember any phone conversation. In fact, he had difficulty remembering the layout of his own house. He didn't know the month or year, and he had no recollection of having entered a political campaign.

Nathan entered a state of complete bewilderment. His loss of memory extended back to events that had occurred five to six months before the explosive telephone conversation with Phil. He couldn't remember from one minute to the next what happened after the call. His wife, panic-stricken, called a doctor for an immediate appointment. I was brought in shortly afterward as a consulting neurologist.

At first I didn't know what to make of Nathan, but as I started to examine him some of his memory faculties slowly but definitely began to return. At the end of two hours, much of his memory had been restored, except that he still had a loss of recent and ongoing memory. He had no recollection of the telephone conversation itself, but he did remember that he was a political candidate and what had happened the previous day.

I thought Nathan might have had a seizure — that perhaps he had been on some tranquilizing medication and had had it withdrawn suddenly. But this was not the case. Blood tests were normal; his neurological examination showed nothing unusual, and a CAT scan of his brain revealed no abnormalities. Furthermore, a computerized brain wave test, which ought to have shown some abnormal slowing if Nathan was in the recovery stages of an epileptic seizure, was absolutely normal.

What was wrong with Nathan? He had a condition known as transient global amnesia, a relatively benign loss of memory in that most persons who experience it recover almost completely and rarely have a recurrence of the problem. What causes it? Some researchers attribute transient global amnesia to a shower of tiny strokes in the memory centers deep in the brain, but no strong evidence supports this theory, and certainly there was no evidence of a stroke in Nathan's case. There was also no sign of a seizure or of any head injury. Nathan had a history of migraine attacks earlier in his life, but he hadn't had one for a long time.

Some neurologists think that transient global amnesia is a rare manifestation of migraine. Perhaps a better explanation of Nathan's case is that so much accumulated stress simply overloaded his neural circuits, which were already sensitized by depression. In fact, it is not uncommon that a history of great and sometimes overwhelming stress just precedes an attack of transient global amnesia.

I believe that stress, particularly overwhelming stress, in a patient who is already depressed may produce severe transient memory loss. The moral of Nathan's experience is not that you should completely avoid all stress, but that your lifestyle should include stress-relieving exercises, which also help dissolve some forms of reactive depression (that is, depression resulting as a reaction to some event).

Most recently, transient global amnesia has been investigated with modern clinical tools such as positron emission tomography (PET scanning). In 1997, French physicians reported on the case of a fifty-nine-year-old woman who suffered from a typical attack of transient global amnesia. PET scans showed reduced oxygen metabolism without reduced blood flow in the left prefrontal and temporal regions, and a reversed pattern over the left occipital cortex. Deeper structures of the brain were also involved. This whole picture was compatible with a migraine-like phenomenon and indicated that the processes involved were more distributed than focal. Of note is the fact that the hippocampus, a part of the brain that is intimately involved in the acquisition of memory, was spared.

Some physicians view transient global amnesia as simply a psychological response to environmental stress. I disagree with this notion. The brains of patients that I have seen with this disorder have been made more susceptible to severe stress by depression. The result of overwhelming stress on such a depressed individual is a brain dysfunction that, although environmental or psychological in its origin, temporarily results in organic brain malfunction. In other words there is actual suppression of brain activity, particularly the brain activity involved in the function of memory. Fortunately, the condition is transient. Patients almost always recover, and recurrence of the problem is rare.

Vital Memory Points to Remember

1. Depression is a very common, and most easily misdiagnosed, reversible cause of memory loss.
2. There are different kinds of depression, all of which cause different degrees of memory loss and each of which requires different kinds of treatment (e.g., psychotherapy for life adjustment problems and medication for neurochemical imbalance).
3. Alcohol may induce a brief euphoria, but it also makes any kind of depression worse.
4. Depression makes one less able to focus attention and concentration and slows memory retrieval.
5. Overwhelming stress may produce severe transient memory loss in persons whose brains have already been incapacitated by depression.
6. Almost all kinds of memory loss associated with depression can be reversed.

7

Other Potential Causes of Reversible Memory Loss

Pain

IN CLINICAL practice, people who experience chronic pain often report problems with memory functioning. A clinical study completed in 1995 of self-reported memory problems was based on two groups of chronic pain patients. Fifty-six patients had pain secondary to automobile accidents; twenty-seven patients suffered pain from various work-related accidents. They were compared to control groups, including twenty-four patients with medical–dental problems and twenty receiving psychotherapy.

The findings of this study indicated that memory complaints were higher in patients with chronic pain than in the medical–dental group or in the psychotherapy patients. No differences were found between patients suffering pain from an automobile accident as compared to patients suffering pain from an industrial accident.

On a questionnaire designed to be specific to memory complaints in chronic pain patients, differences in memory complaints for pain patients as contrasted to controls were found, even after the effects due to depression were statistically removed. There was no report of memory problems attributable to medication.

This study was not unique or really that surprising. People with chronic pain find it difficult to concentrate. They are easily distracted and, as a result, the encoding of messages in the memory center is interfered with. The treatment of this kind of memory disorder has to be directed toward relieving the chronic pain.

Unfortunately, in some people, this is more easily said than done. The important point to remember, however, is that chronic pain can interfere with the memory process. People who suffer chronic pain and who have difficulty functioning efficiently in the workplace may have a memory problem that reduces their functional abilities. This does not mean, however, that they have a structural defect or serious disease of the brain.

Insomnia, Sleep Deprivation, and Brain Anoxia

Lack of oxygen supply to the brain (anoxia) can produce a wide array of brain disabilities. Carbon monoxide poisoning, for example, when it is severe enough to require hospitalization, often produces partial loss of memory function, persisting for some time after the acute poisoning. In a similar fashion, the disease called fatal familial insomnia produces an early impairment of attention, memory deficits (mainly in working memory), and a progressive dream-like state with confusion. Fortunately this is a very rare condition. More common, however, is the sleep apnea syndrome, as studied in a group of veterans of the Persian Gulf war. Sleep apnea is a condition in which people, during periods of sleep, stop breathing because of an obstruction in the upper portion of the airway. This can cause heart problems, including pulmonary hypertension. The chief symptoms of this syndrome include memory loss and fatigue.

People with chronic insomnia perform worse than normal controls on reaction times, they sway more on balance tests, and they forget more numbers on digit span tests. A number of paradoxes are apparent in the assessment and treatment of insomnia and the sleep state. These include the misperception regarding sleep quality and quantity. People with insomnia frequently identify themselves as having been awake when awakened from sleep. They also tend to overestimate sleep latency and underestimate their total sleep time. They appear to derive more subjective benefit from drugs than can be explained by objective measurements.

The depth of sleep is often measured objectively by EEG (electroencephalographic) recordings. Some people who claimed they have not slept at all are by objective EEG measurements in a light stage of sleep. Studies of these people, when they do not have sleep apnea, show no loss of memory function.

A series of 1,500 people, ages thirty to sixty, with habitual snoring and sleep apnea were studied by other researchers. The objective was to evaluate the relationship between snoring and sleep apnea on the one hand and concentration and memory complaints on the other. The main conclusion drawn was that intellectual complaints show a high correlation to mood, insomnia, and hypersomnia (excessive sleep). Habitual snoring and sleep apnea showed a positive correlation to poor concentration, but long-term memory was not affected. The Danish physicians who carried out this study suggested that the association between snoring, sleep apnea, and intellectual loss was related to the presence of sleep disturbances and daytime sleepiness.

Obviously, good sleep habits are conducive to good intellectual function and good memory performance. In the absence of brain disease, medications and drugs do not seem to improve memory, even if they induce sleep. In addition, some of these sleep-producing drugs are habit-forming. Even though it is difficult to develop conditioned reflexes that lead to normal sleep, it is important to train yourself with relaxation exercises, as described in other parts of this book. If these are used effectively, good sleep habits will ensue.

Post-traumatic Stress Disorder

Impaired memory test performance related to post-traumatic stress can reflect a host of factors, such as head injury/post-concussion syndrome, involvement in litigation, malingering, psychological distress, and the use of certain medications. The claim of memory loss in litigation always has to be verified by scrupulous investigation. However, there are certain litigation claims regarding memory loss associated with post-traumatic stress disorder that may have merit.

Attention and memory performances were studied in Persian Gulf war veterans, with and without the diagnosis of post-traumatic stress disorder. Veterans diagnosed with post-traumatic stress disorder showed relative performance deficiencies on tasks of sustained attention, mental manipulation, initial acquisition of information, and retroactive interference.

The patterns of intellectual and memory loss in veterans with post-traumatic stress disorder suggests that the intrusive memories of the traumatic events themselves may be augmented over a period of time by conditioning. Finally, a number of seemingly unrelated environmental stimuli may trigger the flashbacks that produce a disorganization of memory and other intellectual functions.

Another study of post-traumatic stress disorder focused on rape victims. Fifteen rape victims with and sixteen rape victims without post-traumatic stress disorder were tested for learning and memory abilities. The subjects with post-traumatic stress disorder performed significantly worse than the other group. Their performance could be improved to some extent by cues and recognition testing. The memory deficits described in this study were mild and were not attributable to depression, anxiety, or substance abuse.

Obviously, the best way to treat memory deficiency in people with post-traumatic stress disorder is to treat the disorder itself. This is sometimes difficult and tedious, but there are established psychotherapeutic techniques for it.

8

Alcoholism, Brain Poisoning, and Memory Loss

Do you drink an alcoholic beverage every day? Has anyone ever told you that you drink too much? Do you have problems remembering things that are important to you? Have you ever had gaps in your memory, especially after drinking heavily — times that you can't seem to remember what went on, whether for a few hours or even days? Do you find that your memory isn't as sharp now as it was six months or a year ago? If you answered yes to any of these questions, the amount of alcohol you're drinking may be affecting your memory.

This is not to say that anyone who has an occasional (that is, once a month) glass of wine or other alcoholic drink will be irrevocably brain-damaged. But especially if your diet is insufficient or poorly balanced, if you drink every day and feel that your memory abilities are slipping, there are a few facts you need to know. First and foremost, alcohol is a poison.

Alcohol Poisoning

Alcohol poisons the brain and uniformly depresses brain function. The first area of the brain to be affected by alcohol is the limbic or emotional area of the brain. This was originally shown by J. C. Lee, a Canadian scientist who studied the

111

breakdown of the blood–brain barrier in experimental animals after intravascular administration of various amounts of alcohol.

Under ordinary circumstances the blood–brain barrier is a barrier around the capillaries in the brain which prevents unwanted substances from getting into brain cells. But if something disrupts its ability to block substances from entering brain cells, dramatic things can happen in the brain, such as excessive accumulation of ions and chemicals around the cells. Normally the blood–brain barrier keeps ions and chemicals at proper proportions and concentrations for healthy brain function. Calcium ions, for example, are a normal component of the nerve cell environment, but if the blood–brain barrier ceases to operate effectively the consequent buildup of calcium ions can cause brain cell death.

The blood–brain barrier can be broken down by such traumas as brain injury, hemorrhage, tumors, infection, and extreme alteration of the ratio of oxygen to carbon dioxide in the blood that reaches the brain. Alcohol in the blood stream also breaks down the barrier. Significant amounts break down the barrier throughout the entire brain; small amounts break it down only in the limbic brain — the inner parts of the temporal lobes, known as the hippocampus and the amygdala, and the midline parts of the brain, the thalamus and hypothalamus.

One effect of this poisoning of the limbic brain is that the inhibitory restraints that generally govern social conduct and interpersonal relationships are lifted. You have only to stand outside the door of a room where a cocktail party is in progress to measure this breakdown of the blood–brain barrier and the initial poisoning of the emotional brain in the people who are drinking inside. You can hear it. As the limbic brains of more and more of the participants are poisoned, voices become louder and more shrill and the noise of the party increases to a crescendo. After a while, when people's brains become more thoroughly poisoned, the depressing effects of alcohol become apparent and the partygoers become sleepy. If they drink enough, they can even become unconscious.

During the initial phase of brain poisoning, when the inhibitory centers are depressed, persons consuming alcohol do not feel that they have lost intellectual ability. Many people feel slightly elated and grossly overestimate their abilities, including their faculty of memory as well as other intellectual capacities. There may be a very short-term effect initially which makes it appear to individuals that they're able to concentrate better than they could before they began drinking. They often feel they can focus attention on whatever they're doing without the distractions from the outside world which normally worry them or the difficulties stemming from the past which make them less able to function. But this brief period of elation, which is associated with a lack of concern for real-world problems and of capacity for reality testing, quickly passes into a state of general unconcern in which all phases of the memory process are depressed.

Alcohol Poisoning and Memory Loss

Chronic alcohol abuse can produce memory loss in different ways. As people drink, the focusing of attention becomes more difficult, acquisition of new information can be retarded, the memory traces stored are more shallow, and the rate of forgetting of new memories is increased. In addition, the retrieval of memories from the memory bank is also slowed down, and accompanying this increased retrieval time is greater difficulty reconstituting memories. All intellectual functions are diminished. Finally, new memories are simply not elaborated. Many people who drink steadily over a period of hours or days are left with blank spots in their memories in place of a record of what happened during the period of their intoxication — the so-called "lost weekend," named after the forties film.

113

Memory deficits in people who consume large amounts of alcohol are often difficult to ascribe to one cause to the exclusion of others. While it is true that people drinking alcohol are poisoning their brains, other factors may enter the clinical picture, making the precise cause of memory loss difficult to define. Nutritional deficiencies, for example, are common among persons who consume large amounts of alcohol (perhaps 6 percent of the adult population; 10 percent of those who drink alcohol can be classified as alcohol abusers or alcoholics). Certain B vitamins are often lacking in the diets of alcohol abusers, especially vitamin B-1, or thiamine. Thiamine deficiency is associated with a disease called Korsakoff's psychosis, which produces a memory loss and can be corrected only if the thiamine and vitamins B-5 and B-6 are taken in sufficient quantities to saturate the tissue before permanent brain damage occurs.

Repeated or chronic use of alcohol in intoxicating quantities is also associated with brain injury because drunken people tend to fall down and get into accidents. Closed-head injuries often damage the undersurface of the frontal lobes and the anterior parts of the temporal lobes, the area of the brain where the acquisition of new memories occurs.

During the withdrawal stage, alcoholism can bring on epileptic seizures, another cause of memory loss since seizures often begin in the inner part of the temporal lobes in the centers closely related to the acquisition of new memories. Alcoholic seizure, or a "rum fit," is one of the most frequently cited reasons for patients' being admitted to city hospitals.

All of these factors may operate in patients who take in large amounts of alcohol. In some people who are very susceptible, even small amounts of alcohol can have the same effects. For example, a person with any kind of brain injury or brain tumor may set off a train of epileptic seizures with only one or two drinks. My advice to patients with brain tumors, strokes, or injuries is not to drink at all.

Another aspect of the effects of drinking is that many persons who abuse alcohol do so in a vain effort to treat underlying depression. The depression has already reduced certain memory abilities, and of course the use of the alcohol only exacerbates tendencies toward impaired memory function.

Some physicians and brain researchers believe that the effects of alcohol on the brain are really the result of vitamin deficiencies, brain injury, or epileptic seizures related to the use of alcohol. My own experience, however, does not bear this out. Alcohol poisoning by itself, even in healthy persons who have normal diets, produces a decrease in brain function and changes in the structure of the brain. Alterations in the soft tissue of the brain can easily be seen on CAT scans, which reveal a falling away or diminution of some tissues deep inside the brain with a corresponding expansion of spinal fluid into the vacated spaces. These spaces, or lateral ventricles, become very large at times but will often shrink when the alcoholic patient stops drinking.

Alcohol Abuse and Loss of Vital Memory

Chronic alcohol abuse can also produce a loss of intellectual faculties, including a loss of vital memory. The following case may seem like an extreme example, but in many ways it illustrates how alcohol can impair vital memory; in fact, the case of Kenny, one of our patients, was typical of this syndrome.

Before I saw Kenny he had been drinking excessively for years, to the point that he had difficulty even in performing the everyday activities of life. Unless he had the supervision of his wife, his behavior was so unpredictable that his own safety was threatened. Walking in Boston, for example, he would step out into a flow of fast-moving traffic. He didn't recognize his peril in such circumstances, even when he was comparatively sober. In other words, Kenny had lost vital memory about the danger of getting in the way of fast-moving cars; he had lost essential parts of his memory which would keep him out of harm's way.

You may think that there was something peculiar about Kenny — that he didn't eat well or had always been lazy. But before he started drinking too much Kenny had had a good job, and his wife was devoted to him. Even after his heavy drinking began, his wife made sure he ate nutritious meals. Nevertheless, Kenny developed a swelling of the fluid-filled spaces in his brain, with shrinkage of deep tissues. The swellings indicated structural brain damage caused by excessive alcohol intake.

My impression that chronic alcohol abuse causes deteriorating brain function has been confirmed by psychologists like Nelson Butters and his associates. Butters found that alcoholics with adequate nutrition who abstained from all alcoholic beverages still performed well below average in certain learning tasks requiring good recent-memory function. Alcoholics suffering a decrease in their short-term verbal memory were less able to recognize famous faces and did less well than normal controls on tests of recall, a function that dropped off still further among older alcoholic subjects.

Although chronic alcoholics scored substantially lower than normal controls, they still did better than Korsakoff's patients, who have the added problem of vitamin B-1 deficiency. This fact indicates to me that even though thiamine deficiency interrupts memory functions, particularly recent memory, much more powerfully than chronic alcoholism alone, the brain poisoning caused by long-term alcohol abuse plays a role in persistent and progressive memory loss, even after the patient has stopped drinking.

Myths of Alcohol Consumption

No one is immune to the effects of alcohol, and no one is protected from its dangerous side effects. The case history of Kenny may lead you to think that you're in trouble only if you're an alcohol abuser with severely impaired brain function. But that's not true. In one experiment, for example, we tested the neurological function of clergymen who drank frequently but in most other ways were performing normally. Because of their institutional setting these persons' nutrition was excellent, and because of their calling they had superior intellectual ability. Even so, our subjects exhibited decreases in mental function and some aspects of memory. Many of them, who had regularly consumed moderate amounts of alcohol, showed a loss of tissue in the medial part of the frontal lobes, resulting in a widening of the fissure between the two cerebral hemispheres and a decrease in brain tissue in the inner part of the frontal lobes. Long-term alcohol use, we thus concluded, even by well-nourished individuals, produces structural changes in the brain.

The most important fact you should know about alcohol is that it is a brain poison; it disturbs normal brain function. People use it, as they have for millennia, as a shield from the harsh realities of everyday existence. The occasional person, such as Winston Churchill, may abuse alcohol and still be very productive. But for every person who is so fortunate as to escape the long-term results of alcohol poisoning, there are thousands of others who suffer its deleterious effects. Alexander the Great, whose epileptic seizures were probably exacerbated by his abuse of alcohol, and whose premature death at age thirty-three was probably related to his immoderate drinking, is a well-documented historical example.

But without enumerating the famous or infamous persons whose lives were destroyed by alcohol, I want to stress that the average individual who poisons his or her brain with alcohol is less able to solve the problems one encounters from day to day in our competitive and complex society. Memory impairment by brain poisoning makes us less prepared and less resourceful in responding to the challenges of our world.

My own view is that for optimal brain function the intake of alcohol should be zero. I base my opinion on data recorded during Prohibition, when as a nation we tried the social experiment of trying to eliminate all alcohol consumption. The experiment failed because of the corruption and greed of the public officials responsible for managing it. Nevertheless, Prohibition was a conspicuous medical success. The years during which the manufacture and sale of alcohol were outlawed in the United States saw a great reduction in deaths from cirrhosis of the liver and an even more striking decrease in the number of admissions to state mental hospitals for alcohol-related psychosis. We'll undoubtedly never return to prohibition in this country, but the data prove conclusively that reduced alcohol consumption benefits health.

I am always asked about those over fifty who take a drink to improve digestion. Alcohol does stimulate the stomach's secretion of hydrochloric acid (which is why it is bad for people with ulcers). But other gastric stimulants for persons whose secretion of hydrochloric acid is deficient can be prescribed by a physician once such a diagnosis has been confirmed.

Finally, there is the question of the celebratory glass of wine taken once a month or once a week. How much harm will a single glass of wine or can of beer do to the brain? The answer is that we don't know. If a person seldom drinks, having a glass of wine or beer at parties perhaps four or five times a year, the chances are that such a small level of consumption will have a negligible effect. Drinking beer or wine every day, however, is potentially harmful to brain cells. And as an individual progresses from beer or wine to whiskey or cocktails, the effects become definitely harmful.

The common denominator is not what kind of alcoholic beverage is drunk but how much alcohol is getting to the brain. On average, heavier people tolerate alcohol better than thin people and men better than women. Also, some individuals have more protective enzymes to detoxify alcohol than others. Once alcohol gets to the brain in sufficient concentrations, however, it is poisonous. The important issues are the intensity of the poison, the duration of its effects, and how healthy one's brain is to begin with. Even drinking a lot of beer can severely poison your brain, although the proportion of alcohol in each glass is small.

Recently there have been a number of reports indicating a reduction in the incidence of coronary disease in people who consume four or five glasses of alcohol per week. Associated with this is the finding in these test subjects of a slight increase in high-density lipoproteins. There are also some reports indicating that red wine is more beneficial than other alcoholic beverages, but the evidence is inconclusive. Without question, however, whatever beneficial effect alcohol consumption confers is reversed if the number of alcoholic drinks exceeds four or five a week.

Some, but not all, of these cardiac benefits can be duplicated by large amounts of red grape juice. Furthermore, there are other substances, such as aspirin, vitamin E, and other antioxidants associated with dietary changes and exercise, that will give an even more beneficial effect in terms of reducing coronary disease.

Some big questions remain regarding the exact effect of alcohol on high-density lipoproteins. It turns out that there are several types of high-density lipoproteins, and elevation of only one of these is associated with a reduction in coronary artery disease. The exact effect of alcohol in this regard has not been completely determined.

There are preliminary reports that a few drinks of alcohol a week will reduce the incidence of nonhemorrhagic strokes. On the other hand there is some evidence that alcohol intake will increase the incidence of brain hemorrhage. (We will discuss this subject in greater detail later in the section on strokes.)

Leaving aside the discussion of potential cardiovascular benefits, the evidence relating alcohol brain poisoning to memory impairment is very substantial. While there have been a few reports in the literature that moderate daily alcohol use has not decreased memory performance, a more comprehensive study has shown that the memory performance that is relatively preserved in alcoholics includes only the most rudimentary or simple memory functions. On the other hand, there is no question that complex memory functions are severely impaired. Among other things, the alcoholics in the study had a disruption of the executive processes of their brain, especially those processes necessary for coping with complex tasks.

Among the often overlooked consequences of alcohol intake is the effect that this drug has on the brain when it is combined with other drugs. For example, a study of nurses who were dependent upon alcohol and the sedative meperidine showed that they experienced memory loss or memory blackouts while at work. The combination of alcohol and benzodiazepines (sedatives) in an experimental study showed impaired spatial memory. This impairment was related to the reduction of certain neurotransmitters in the dorsal hippocampus.

The choice is yours to make. Your brain is the most precious organ in your body. It needs the utmost protection — especially from brain poisons. All of us often balance, whether consciously or not, the pleasure a particular behavior gives us against the risks. When you drink you know about the pleasure, but you may think that the only risk you face is a hangover. Unfortunately, continual use of alcohol may have long-term adverse consequences on your memory and thought processes, consequences that are not completely reversible even when you stop drinking. The sad fact is that you may not even be aware of your loss until some novel challenge or emergency arises which requires you to make the nice judgment or the right choice that your brain is no longer capable of making. In other words, you may not realize how much damage you've done until it's too late to fix it.

You may have to change your lifestyle, such as by cutting out the nightly cocktail or beer you have while watching television, or not having that glass of wine at every social gathering you attend. It may ultimately mean a reevaluation of the balance between pleasure and pain. If you're in doubt as to where you stand, perhaps you should have a detailed neuropsychological test performed to see if you are slipping mentally and therefore need to reduce or eliminate alcohol from your diet.

Vital Memory Points to Remember

1. Alcohol is related to 10 percent of all deaths in the United States each year.
2. Alcohol is a tissue poison that acts on the limbic area of the brain.
3. Even small amounts of alcohol break down the blood–brain barrier.
4. Joining an organization such as Alcoholics Anonymous is a good first step in helping you control a drinking problem.

9

The Effects of Stimulants, Depressants, and Drugs That Produce Hallucinations on Memory and Intelligence

MOST OF US during our lives experiment with drugs by drinking alcohol or using coffee, tea, or tobacco. Some of us experiment with marijuana, cocaine, speed, or even heroin. While I don't equate the use of coffee or tobacco with that of speed or heroin, all these agents have something in common: they affect and even poison the limbic portion of our brains. If they didn't have such an effect hardly anyone would use them. And, of course, our memory functions are centered in the limbic brain and are influenced in one way or another by all of these drugs.

Some people get hooked on street drugs quite innocently. Some heroin abusers began as patients with chronic pain who were given long-term medical treatment with narcotics. Some people who abuse speed were prescribed diet pills by their physicians which contained a speedlike component, and they became hooked on amphetamines. The chronic use of these drugs not only made them amphetamine-dependent but also produced personality changes, including mood disturbances and paranoia. Many of these persons develop cross dependencies on other street drugs and alcohol as well.

The point is that all street drugs, when used frequently over a long period of time, have bad effects on the brain, including depression, craving for drugs, reduced memory and intellectual abilities, and epileptic seizures. Also, these effects may linger after drug use has been discontinued and crop up months and even years later, which indicates the long-term deleterious effects of many of these agents.

Stimulants

In addition to patients who inadvertently became hooked on amphetamines by taking diet pills, I've met many people in my medical practice who take stimulants to "improve" thinking and memory or just to feel better and be more energetic. They get an initial lift in feeling and mental prowess, but it doesn't last. And using amphetamines and speed over and over produces just the opposite of the results they wanted. This happened to Jerry, who should have known better because he was a medical student.

Jerry was twenty-five years old, had an attractive smile, and was quite popular. But although I considered him to be a bright young man, I knew he thought of himself as an underachiever. That's because Jerry tested very low on standard intelligence tests, and his scores on the college aptitude boards were so inferior that he was not able to gain admission to a regular college but had to go to a remedial one until he showed he could keep up the quality of work necessary in college studies.

That he did well enough not only to graduate from college but also to be admitted to medical school was a surprise to both him and his parents. But he never believed he had accomplished this on his own. He thought his performance in medical school depended on his use of a chemical stimulant, an amphetamine-like drug that fell in the category of street drugs known as speed.

In small amounts this drug did speed up his mental processes, allowing him to focus more intensely on the subjects he was studying and to retain the information well

123

enough to pass tests. But then he forgot everything he had learned very quickly and had to start all over again for the next examination.

Over a period of time Jerry found that he couldn't achieve the same scholastic results with the small amount of stimulant he had been using, and so of course he increased the dose. With the increased dose, however, he was distressed to find that his powers of concentration didn't improve, but got worse. He became agitated and hyperdistractible, he couldn't concentrate, and he wasn't able to focus his attention with enough intensity to retain the material he had to learn to pass his examinations. As a result, his grades began to fall off. His performance as a student deteriorated to the point that he was failing some of his courses and just barely passing others. Jerry also began to undergo personality changes, becoming rather suspicious and at times aggressive.

The sad part of Jerry's story is that he did have the ability to be a satisfactory student without using mind-altering drugs. This realization grew on him only very slowly, and at great personal cost. In the interim, Jerry learned with much anguish his lesson about the addictive nature of stimulants.

The story has a happy ending: Jerry finally got himself off drugs and graduated from medical school — but just barely. He went on to pass his medical boards and became a competent physician.

The effects that stimulants had on Jerry are not unusual. The initial dose, particularly if it is small, will often enhance memory function and increase concentration; it also brings about some elevation of mood, which also helps in focusing attention. As the dose is increased, however, the three elements of memory, acquisition, storage, and retrieval, begin to deteriorate, and performance, particularly with regard to new learning, is diminished.

Ingesting excessive amounts of these medications can produce an acute confusional state marked by disorientation and even hallucinations. Meaningful memory testing is often impossible in these circumstances. Some neurological purists doubt that memory loss occurs in this state because significant testing can't be done. My view, however, is that vital memory is always lost in confusional states characterized by disorientation. In other words, if you don't know where or who you are or what the year or season is, your vital memory is seriously impaired.

Repeated use of stimulants only enhances their negative effects. The elevation of mood proceeds too far, to hyperexcitability, which in turn leads to distraction, not concentration, and consequent difficulty in acquiring new information for storage in the memory bank.

Special considerations must be applied in the self-administration of various illegal stimulants because they are sometimes used to reverse the symptoms of underlying depression. The results are uniformly disappointing, and sometimes dangerous.

Cocaine is often used for this purpose, especially if the depression is of the bipolar variety called manic-depressive illness. All too often the euphoria produced by a dose of cocaine is followed by a depression that is much worse than the original one. The anxiety and hyperactivity associated with cocaine effects, however, may not disappear even when the rebound depression is full-blown. Of course the effects on every aspect of memory, concentration, and new learning are devastating. As with amphetamines, cocaine can also lead to states of increased suspiciousness and even paranoid delusions.

Some cocaine users go on to become aggressive and even dangerous in initiating unprovoked attack behavior. Their memories are selectively and sometimes randomly inhibited during these episodes, and they may not remember their actions afterward. Cocaine can also provoke epileptic seizures or start the kindling of epileptic seizures in the emotional brain. Such abnormal electrical activity is so close to the memory circuits that it may severely disrupt memory function. Cocaine use can also produce devastating changes in the blood vessels of the brain and heart.

The stimulant drugs that are very closely related to amphetamines, such as methylamphetamine, can cause lasting disturbances in brain function in terms of decreasing memory abilities. Almost all the stimulant-type drugs are dangerous as far as memory and brain integrity are concerned, both functionally and structurally. Related compounds like Ritalin, however, are used therapeutically in hyperactive children with minimal brain damage and have the paradoxical effect of calming them down and improving their ability to retain new information. But even Ritalin has unwanted effects on the brains of normal people, and a substantial amount of medical controversy still swirls around the use of this agent.

Coffee, Tea, and Tobacco

Coffee, tea, and tobacco are the most common brain stimulants, although of a much milder sort. The use of tobacco has the most ominous health effects of the three not only because of the carcinogenic potential of tars and nicotine and their action in provoking abnormalities in the lungs, blood vessels, and heart but also because nicotine is intensely addictive.

Many people who drink coffee think that it helps them concentrate. A recent study of the effects of caffeine on healthy college students, however, showed only an insignificant influence on learning and memory performance. A small dose of caffeine decreased boredom and relaxation and increased certain subjective moods such as anxiety, tenseness, and nervousness. Many moderate to frequent users of coffee felt that it helped their recall. In any case, the actual effect of coffee on memory is difficult to assess because the effect is so small.

At a radio station where I was to speak I was recently approached by a young woman employee of the station who asked, in a quiet voice so no one else could hear, whether she could improve her memory and recall for a major examination by drinking a lot of coffee or taking caffeine pills. It was an important test, one that she was concerned about doing well on, and she had heard that drinking coffee while studying and taking the test would improve her performance. I explained that caffeine might confer a minor benefit in that perhaps her attention span would improve, but that she ran the risk of becoming even more agitated, which would ultimately cancel any benefits of better concentration. As unpatronizingly as I could, I gave her my best advice: to study as much as possible and get a good night's sleep before the exam.

Depressants

Sedative drugs, including alcohol, have a marked effect in depressing memory, and the effects are dose-dependent. The higher the blood level of the agent used, the more likely one is to impair all phases of memory function. These agents were originally used medically to combat epileptic seizures. Many years ago, bromides were the drug of choice, but they had so many severe side effects that they were supplanted by the barbiturates. While barbiturates did control some epileptic seizures and the anxiety that surrounded them, they also produced a strong sedative effect. It was once not uncommon, before the advent of Dilantin, to see epileptic patients walk around looking like zombies, barely able to keep their eyes open. Of course, memory function was terribly impaired in this group of patients. Barbiturates were also widely prescribed as sleeping pills and tranquilizers, but the word *sedative* was substituted for *tranquilizer*.

More recently the barbiturates have been supplanted by the so-called minor tranquilizers. Although Valium has a limited use in controlling seizures, this and other agents are chiefly prescribed for their sedative effects. I'm speaking of not only Valium but such drugs as Ativan, Librium, Serax, Xanax, and Atarax. I don't mean to suggest that these agents don't have a place in medicine; they do. Xanax in particular is very useful in treating a certain kind of panic disorder. What I do know is that their role in medicine should be much more circumscribed than is now the case.

Millions of Americans take these drugs, even though many patients don't need them. Almost all of these patients have a degree of impaired memory as a result (if you measure memory abilities after the administration of the drugs and compare them with memory abilities before the drugs were started). Most of these drugs produce substantial memory impairment after the first day of administration. In some cases the impairment may be so severe that whole episodes of the patient's life are forgotten. In some ways this pattern resembles the lost weekend syndrome caused by imbibing large amounts of alcohol, which also depresses brain function.

Elderly persons are often given these tranquilizers to quiet their anxieties, and they are generally more susceptible to their poisonous effects on their memories. Reducing dosage can be therapeutic.

Hallucinogens

Hallucinogenic drugs are taken for no other purpose than to produce hallucinations or visions in the brains of people using them. Some hallucinogenic drugs are synthesized in the laboratory, and the chemist can combine hallucinogens with stimulants to tailor-make a drug to the abuser's wishes, producing a so-called designer drug.

One of the more strikingly effective hallucinogens is LSD-25. This drug, derived from the ergot fungus, was the outcome of the twenty-fifth experiment conducted with the fungus by a Swiss chemist, Dr. A. Hofman. It produces the vivid hallucinations and distortions of time characteristic of all these agents.

One of my psychiatric colleagues at the Massachusetts General Hospital was called on to treat several graduate students in theoretical mathematics at the Massachusetts Institute of

Technology who, after experimenting with LSD, suffered recurring hallucinations after they stopped using the drug. Through prolonged treatment he was able to relieve their immediate symptoms, but he noted over the long term that their intellectual abilities and their memories had deteriorated. These were brilliant, productive people before they started their experimentation with drugs, and they were still smart even after the effects of the drug had worn off. But the use of LSD had decreased their intelligence and their memory abilities slightly yet permanently. Their creative abilities were also somewhat diminished, and many realized they were no longer able to contribute new ideas in their field. The diminution in their abilities was caused by the concentration of this chemical agent in the inner part of the emotional brain, a part called the hippocampus, which produced a deterioration in cells also serving in the memory circuitry. Similar drugs, like PCPs and Angel Dust, do the same thing and often cause epileptic seizures.

One of the most commonly abused hallucinogens in the United States is marijuana. There has been a lot of controversy over whether this agent has deleterious effects on the brain. Extensive studies of the effects of marijuana leave no question that it impairs learning and the retention of new information. In other words, its continued use does undermine memory.

Whether memory loss stemming from marijuana use is permanent or not is difficult to assess because we do not have the necessary psychological evaluations of chronic users of marijuana before they began smoking marijuana, so it is impossible to determine how much their intellectual abilities may have declined after using the drug. It is known, however, that smoking a single marijuana cigarette affects the brain, particularly in slowing reaction times. Of course marijuana, like other drugs — depressants (including tranquilizers), alcohol, stimulants, and hallucinogens — is taken because of its effect on the brain. Even very mild drugs are essentially brain toxins whose effects, even in low doses, result from an alteration or poisoning of brain function.

The central question is how much brain poisoning we can tolerate, and whether the poisoning is worth the feelings we get from having our inhibitions dampened or our moods elevated. Each person must answer this question for him- or herself, but everyone should at least be aware of the harmful effects of these agents in suppressing memory and depressing brain function.

If you want to get off street drugs but can't do it by yourself, you should seek medical help from an addiction program near you. There is often a transference between drug abuse and alcohol abuse, so programs like Alcoholics Anonymous can also be helpful for some patients with drug problems. Don't be reluctant to ask for help, because kicking a drug habit can almost never be accomplished alone.

Vital Memory Points to Remember

1. The repeated use of stimulants tends to diminish memory abilities and capacity for new learning.
2. Cocaine use can cause memory impairment.
3. The actual effect of coffee drinking on memory is hard to assess because the effect is so small.
4. Almost all drugs that alter normal brain function will produce some degree of memory impairment if taken in sufficient quantities over a long enough period of time.

10

Prescription Medications That Cause Memory Loss

ARE YOU TAKING some kind of medication prescribed by your doctor, which you've been on for a long time? Has your dose been changed recently, or have you been given a new medicine, one that you weren't on before? If so, have you noticed any change in your intelligence, memory, or mood since you started the new medicine or changed the amount of your old medicine? Or has there been any recent change in your memory, mood, or mental abilities, even though you haven't started on a new medicine or dosage? This happened to Henry, whose mental changes were related to the doctor-prescribed medicine he was taking.

Henry was a sixty-seven-year-old patient of mine who had severe intermittent abdominal pain. For thirty years he went from one physician to another and had a number of thorough examinations, including special x-ray tests, all of which failed to disclose the reason for his problem. He was finally diagnosed as having spastic bowel syndrome and was put on daily doses of phenobarbital and belladonna. Sometimes these medications worked and sometimes they didn't, but Henry kept taking them for months, and eventually years.

About nine months before I saw him he had begun to become more forgetful, generally duller, and less intellectually reactive to his wife and family. They thought he must be getting Alzheimer's disease, but our tests didn't indicate any specific problems in his brain except for some changes in his brain wave test, which showed difficulty in brain metabolism.

When we examined the medications Henry had been taking, his wife assured me that he had been taking the same dose of each for many years. I was sure that the medications were the villains in causing his memory loss. Belladonna interferes with the brain's use of acetylcholine, the neurotransmitter related to the memory circuits in the inner part of the temporal lobes, whereas phenobarbital is long-acting and its effect tends to accumulate in the central nervous system. I didn't want simply to stop the medications, however, since a patient who has been on phenobarbital for a long time and suddenly stops taking it is very apt to have epileptic seizures.

What I did was gradually reduce the dosages of the medications. Within a few days, the lowered blood level of these drugs resulted in improvement in both Henry's memory and his intellectual function. After three weeks, by then on much-reduced doses, Henry was back to normal functioning and still free of pain.

The lesson to be learned from this case, and many similar ones, is that it isn't always necessary to discontinue someone's medication even though it may be directly related to their symptoms of impaired mental function and memory loss. Henry needed help for his abdominal pain, but that help had to be balanced with the consequences of consuming the medications. Sometimes just reducing the dosage of medication is enough to restore a patient's normal mental function.

One always has to stay alert to this need for balancing. Someone can take a medication at the same dosage for a long period of time without having any noticeable effects on the brain or brain function. Suddenly, when abrupt changes in lifestyle or in the inner chemistry and metabolism of the body (whether or not related to age) occur, the person can no longer tolerate the same dose of medication.

This finding is not unusual, and physicians should be aware of it, although sometimes they aren't. It is true for people of all ages but especially for the elderly, whose bodies can be slower in detoxifying or eliminating medications. Also, as we grow older we have fewer brain cells, and even if these cells function more efficiently, they are more susceptible to brain poisoning because there is less brain reserve. It is more difficult for an older person with fewer brain cells to recover from a serious brain insult, whether caused by brain injury or brain poisoning, than it is for a child, for example, who has many more brain cells.

Doctors certainly know that infants, children, and adults require different dosage schedules of medications. What they often fail to realize is that people over the age of fifty-five, and particularly over sixty, should follow a reduced dosage schedule. And of course, the older people get, the more susceptible they become to side effects from what might have been well-tolerated dosages of medications they took at a younger age, whether the drugs affected the brain or not.

You will notice that I have been focusing on the memory or intellectual changes that follow the use of a new drug or a change in dosage of one of the medicines you are currently taking. Drugs can produce many other kinds of changes, from sleep disturbances to dry mouth or itching. If you have any of these symptoms, it should be called to the attention of your doctor, but I have not discussed such symptoms in detail because they may not be related to your memory problems.

Every drug known has dose-dependent side effects or toxic consequences. A drug's side effects are usually listed by the manufacturer in a statement enclosed in the package. I urge you to read these statements. Unfortunately, many drug companies do not include the adverse effects of their compounds on brain function and memory, an omission I would like to see corrected.

TABLE 1 **Potentially Toxic or Poisonous Prescription Drugs That Commonly Produce Problems with Memory or Intelligence**

Psychiatric Drugs	Drugs Used in General Medicine
Barbiturates	Digitalis preparations
Bromides	Analgesics
Benzodiazepines	Antihypertensives (especially beta blockers)
Phenothiazines	Antidiabetic agents
Haloperidol	Cimetidine
Lithium	Methyldopa
Antidepressants	Inderal
	Reserpine
	Symmetrel
	Drugs with anticholinergic actions (seasickness pills)
	Antihistamines
	Eye drops for glaucoma

Source: Dr. Thomas D. Sabin, Boston City Hospital.

Table 1 is a partial list of drugs that can alter memory and intellectual functions. In addition, certain combinations of drugs — Mellaril and lithium, for example, or haloperidol and methyldopa — are likely to produce confusion and memory loss.

Major Tranquilizers and Memory Loss

In the last chapter we discussed the effects of bromides, barbiturates, and tranquilizers in depressing memory function and decreasing memory abilities. The tranquilizers we discussed were the so-called minor tranquilizers, which are routinely given to people who have agitation or panic attacks.

The major tranquilizers, such as the phenothiazines — including Thorazine, Prolixin, Compazine, Mellaril, and Stelazine — produce much more severe brain dysfunction and memory loss than the minor tranquilizers. These agents (used mainly on profoundly agitated, hallucinating, delusional psychiatric patients) can cause symptoms very much like those of Parkinson's disease: an inability to initiate movement, a masklike facial expression, a shuffling gait, and slowness of movement.

A great number of people who take this kind of drug for a period of time develop a disorder of the central nervous system called tardive dyskinesia. This syndrome, which begins weeks to months after the agent is first administered, consists of involuntary movements of the face or tongue, with occasional tonic spasms of the legs and arms. These complications can occur after even an initial dose of the medication, although that's rare. More often the abnormal movements of the face, tongue, and neck occur late and become persistent complications. Occasionally these agents produce a catatonic rigidity and stupor.

Related drugs like haloperidol (Haldol) have much the same antipsychotic effects as the phenothiazines. They may also have the same kinds of side effects, and they do tend to cause severe interruptions of thought and memory which are oftentimes dose-dependent. Reducing or eliminating this drug will reduce its toxic effects on thinking and memory, but often a decrease in dosage will precipitate a recurrence of the original symptoms, including hallucinations, that first prompted the use of this agent. Of course, the movement disorders described as tardive dyskinesia may persist even after the drug has been completely discontinued.

Antidepressants and Memory Loss

Another class of psychoactive drugs, many of which have different chemical characteristics, are the antidepressants. It is not my purpose to discourage people from using psychoactive drugs if they are necessary in treating psychiatric disease. Severe depression is certainly an indication for their use. It is important to realize, however, that not all psychoactive drugs have the same effects or act through the same mechanisms. This is particularly true with antidepressants, as the following story illustrates.

Molly, a fifty-seven-year-old advertising copywriter who was subject to depression, was referred to me by her psychiatrist when she began to have symptoms of memory loss. She had difficulty performing her complex job because she couldn't keep all the variables and facets of her responsibility in focus. Because of her chronic depression she was taking a drug called Elavil, which had been very effective. More recently her doses of the agent had been slightly increased to give her the same therapeutic effect, and that's when she began to suffer memory loss.

Elavil not only improves the mood; it also has the effect of interfering with the acetylcholine network in the brain. Realizing that Molly needed to be on an antidepressant, I suggested that her psychiatrist change her to Prozac. Not all antidepressants are equally effective in treating the symptoms of a given patient, and there has to be a certain amount of trial and error to see whether the patient will respond to any one of them. Molly had responded to Elavil, and she also responded to Prozac — and this antidepressant was less toxic to Molly's memory function than Elavil.

You should not get the idea from this example that Elavil is not a useful drug and that Prozac is; the effectiveness of any drug depends on the unique biochemistry of each patient. The Prozac relieved Molly's depression and did not impair her memory, although there was no way of knowing what the result of her taking the drug would be before she tried it. (Incidentally, double-blind crossover experiments have shown that Elavil has a slightly greater tendency to impair intellectual and memory functions than does Prozac.) The point in my telling you this story is not to recommend one antidepressant over another, but merely to indicate that it is possible to substitute one medication for another when each has similar therapeutic effects on the user but is tolerated quite differently.

However, there is no perfect antidepressant, though some have fewer side effects than others. Elavil, for example, one of a class of drugs known as the tricyclic antidepressants, often causes people taking it to experience dryness in their mouths, constipation, dizziness (particularly when standing up quickly), weight gain, and sleepiness. Others may experience increased sensitivity to the sun, confusion, and even agitation. Prozac, even though it is generally thought to produce fewer side effects, can bring about nervousness, diarrhea, headaches, drowsiness, and insomnia, depending on the individual. Before you take either of these drugs — or any drug, for that matter — it's always wise to know as much about the possible long- and short-term side effects as you can.

The treatment of people who have been brain-poisoned by one medication is not simply to take them off all medications; doing so would also deprive them of needed therapy. Rather, the solution is to carefully titrate and adjust the dosage of the medication causing the problem, and if that doesn't work then to shift medications cautiously to try to find one that works without producing toxicity.

Monitoring Potentially Dangerous Situations

Certain combinations of drugs, like Mellaril and lithium or haloperidol and the antihypertensive drug methyldopa, are known to be particularly likely to produce memory loss and other forms of intellectual deterioration and even a confusional state. Also, a number of medicines that supposedly have nothing to do with the brain can cause rather pronounced alteration of mental function or loss of memory. This is why it's important to have a single knowledgeable physician to monitor all the medications you take — not just psychiatric or brain medications but also medications for the heart, lungs, kidneys, and so on. Your doctor must make sure that you are not becoming intoxicated or, in particular, brain-poisoned. This physician may have to contact your other specialists if a change in medications is necessary so that important drug therapies are not disturbed.

If you don't have a single physician monitoring your medications, it is possible that each of the specialists you see will write a prescription for a drug to treat one or another part of your body. You might end up with a heart medication, glaucoma medication, antihypertensive medication, and then possibly a sedative. All of these medications may affect your brain function and specifically your memory. Sometimes the combination of drugs is more poisonous to your brain than a single drug alone. Psychiatrists who specialize in psychopharmacology may be able to measure the toxic effects of all of the agents you take. But if a psychiatrist is your principal physician, he or she must be in communication with your other doctors and be aware of other prescription medications you take which are not associated with the brain but can impair brain function and memory.

Antihypertensive Drugs and Memory Loss

Just as with the antidepressant drugs, antihypertensive agents may have various effects on memory and intellectual capacity. Again, this phenomenon is individualized. Antihypertensive agents that are beta blockers, like propranolol and atenolol, may decrease memory performance more consistently than antihypertensive agents that act through a different mechanism, such as angiotensin-converting enzyme inhibitors like enalapril, which have very little effect on memory. (Angiotensin is a hormone involved in controlling arterial pressure.)

Some of the drugs that can impair memory include digitalis

preparations, drugs to relieve pain, antihypertensive agents (as we've discussed), and any agent that depresses the level of blood glucose, especially those for treatment of diabetes. Eye drops for glaucoma, and even gastrointestinal drugs like cimetidine, may produce a loss of memory and interfere with other intellectual functions.*

Polypharmacy

It's always a challenge to go into a nursing home to review a patient who has had a recent decrease in memory abilities and intellectual function. Of course, after ruling out obvious physical problems that may affect the brain, I always try to find out whether the person has had a recent depression or change in mood. Next I look at the medications the patient is on. Often I am dismayed because many patients were started on several medications and, as time went by, one medication was added to another, with none of them ever stopped. This is what we call polypharmacy.

Jim, a retired mechanic who came to see me from Connecticut, was such a patient. He had a long list of the medications he took, and the doctors who prescribed these medicines weren't particularly concerned about their effects on the brain because none of the drugs were primarily for brain problems. And yet Jim had an obvious decrease in memory abilities and intellectual capacity from the combined effects of all these medications. It was then a matter of trial and error in slowly decreasing the dosages of those drugs that might be inessential to see if we could uncover the guilty culprit or culprits — that is, the drug or combination of drugs that had such a toxic effect on Jim's brain function.

*A relevant case here is that of former President Bush, who was diagnosed in early 1990 as having a mild case of glaucoma in one eye for which eye drops were prescribed. Shortly after making the diagnosis, his doctors put him on the new medication but they quickly took him off it, possibly because they realized that the drops might adversely affect his judgment or memory.

In Jim's case it turned out to be three different medications: one for his heart, one for his high blood pressure, and one for asthma. What my associates and I tried to do was cut out those medications that could be dispensed with and substitute others at lower dosages to treat the medical conditions that required continuous therapy. Obviously we were not so zealous in reducing his medication that he would develop any symptoms of undertreated disease.

Besides his supportive family, Jim had a cooperative and concerned physician who had initially referred him to our Center for Memory Impairment. His doctor began to carry out our recommendations — slowly, in order to avoid the toxic effects of abrupt withdrawal of medications. At the same time, he substituted medications that were less toxic to Jim than the ones he had been taking. After Jim's third trip to the Center for Memory Impairment, he was dramatically improved without suffering any side effects because appropriate medications had been substituted to treat his heart condition, his high blood pressure, and his asthma.

Antiemetics and Seasickness Medications

I'd like to say a word to all the sailors reading this who have a tendency to get seasick. Some people who are prone to motion sickness often use transdermal patches applied behind their ears which infuse a medication that masks the symptoms of *mal de mer*. If the medication is scopolamine, they'd better be cautious about sailing because this drug can have a negative effect on memory and other intellectual functions.

At one time, particularly in the late twenties, women in the throes of childbirth were often given large doses of scopolamine. This drug was prescribed because it didn't inhibit uterine contractions and at the same time was supposed to make the women more comfortable. Actually it didn't do much for their comfort. But when they were questioned after the event, they had very few complaints about how their obstetrical management was handled. In fact, they had no memory of the event at all; the scopolamine had completely wiped out their memories. This phenomenon, then known as "twilight sleep," resulted from an interference with the acetylcholine mechanisms in the hippocampus which are essential in acquiring new memories.

Scopolamine has such a profound effect in reducing memory function that it is often used in a wide variety of medical experiments. But you should be aware that any agent used to reduce nausea or vertigo, and especially seasickness, may also have the tendency to adversely affect memory function. If you sail, you might not be able to make accurate nautical measurements and exercise superior seamanship and judgment if your memory circuits — those parts of the brain which are so necessary to any intellectual process — are working at half speed or less.

How and When to Talk to Your Doctor

The most important lesson you can draw from this chapter is that of the necessity of self-reliance. In the final analysis, it is you who consumes the prescription drugs, and it is you who must be responsible for preventing drug-induced impairment of your mind or memory. Your best safeguard against self-inflicted damage is to question your doctor carefully every time a new drug is prescribed or the dose is changed on one you are already taking. Your questions should include the following:

1. Why am I taking this drug?
2. Why do I need this drug?
3. Why is the dose being changed?
4. What are the toxic effects of this drug?
5. What are the effects of taking this drug for a long time?

6. Will this drug interfere with any other drug I'm taking?
7. Will this drug combine with another drug I'm taking to be more toxic than either alone?
8. Will this drug affect my mind or my memory?
9. How long will I be on this drug?
10. What toxic effects might arise if I discontinue taking this drug?

Remember, it is your life and brain function that are at stake. You deserve courteous and complete answers to your questions, and if you don't get them you may need another doctor.

Vital Memory Points to Remember

1. As we get older, our functioning brain cells decrease in number and become more susceptible to brain poisoning.
2. There should be reduced dosage schedules of medications for people over age fifty-five.
3. Major tranquilizers can produce severe memory loss.
4. Some antidepressants may cause memory loss.
5. A single physician should be in charge of monitoring all your prescriptions in order to reduce the possibility of adverse side effects from their combination.

Diet and Reversible Memory Loss

YOUR BRAIN is a very sensitive organ requiring precise amounts of sugar, oxygen, water, sodium, potassium, and vitamins in order to function properly. If there isn't enough sugar or oxygen, or there's too much water, or insufficient nutrition (such as a lack of certain key vitamins), your brain function and especially your memory can deteriorate dramatically.

Many possible reasons can account for imbalances in our brains' support systems as we grow older. For example, with advancing age we are often less active. We therefore eat smaller amounts of food since we need fewer calories. That's not bad if with the decreased amount of food we receive sufficient vitamins, especially B vitamins. But for those of us who don't supplement our diets with vitamin pills this may not be the case. Good diets of 1,800 to 2,200 calories a day may not contain enough essential thiamine (vitamin B-1), for example, to replenish body stores, and vitamin B deficiencies may occur, particularly in times of stress.

Another reason we may not get enough B vitamins as we grow older is that we may lose teeth and not be able to chew food properly for thorough digestion of nutrients. And of course, if we have poor teeth, we are going to avoid foods we have to chew and take foods that are semisolid and go down

143

easily. These foods may not contain enough B vitamins or even proteins.

In Chapter 11 I discuss only briefly what happens when all the nutrients obtained from the diet are reduced to dangerously low levels. Fortunately, such malnutrition is rare in the United States except in certain pockets of extreme poverty. The majority of the chapter describes the more likely scenario, namely an inadequate intake of some of the important B vitamins.

Chapter 12 describes some aspects of brain chemistry, focusing on concentrations of certain electrolytes and water which affect memory. The balancing of these substances is especially significant to us as we grow older since if we don't take in proper amounts of water and electrolytes during hot and humid days our brain function can be impaired.

Chapter 13 focuses on problems of memory that stem from a relative lack of oxygen and sugar in the arterial blood stream, and in turn in the capillary blood bringing oxygen and sugar to the brain cells. Chapter 14 discusses thyroid dysfunction.

So many mechanisms and controls have to work perfectly in order to keep intelligence and memory performing at optimal levels that it often seems a wonder our brains work as well as they do. To regulate these complicated processes, the human body has a series of checks and balances which in a delicate, sophisticated, and accurate way feed information back to control centers. These centers are part of the early warning, failsafe mechanisms that usually prevent abnormalities from occurring and ensure that the brain, the most important organ in our bodies, is given top priority, along with the heart and lungs, in any stressful situation. Disease, injury, and chronic neglect can break down these fail-safe mechanisms, however, and cause intellectual and memory functions to decline. Understanding how some of these important mechanisms work will help us avoid potentially dangerous pitfalls.

11

Memory Loss Related to Brain Nutrition

Is YOUR DIET adequate, or do you eat junk foods that are high in fat and loaded with salt? Can you chew your food properly, or are your teeth in such poor condition (or your plates so loose) that you give up on foods that need to be chewed thoroughly before they can be swallowed? Are you a food faddist, adopting the latest diet to lose weight and then rapidly gaining it all back, only to go on another crazy diet again, perhaps one requiring liquid protein supplements? Do you find that your appetite is fading and that you are eating less and less food?

If you fall into any of these categories you may have a nutritional deficiency that can affect your memory. A number of nutritional deficiency problems can alter vital memory, even in those of us who are generally not malnourished or protein-starved. For example, a deficiency in minerals like calcium, phosphorus, iodine, iron, magnesium, copper, or zinc can undermine mental functions. Also, the water-electrolyte balance must be kept in proper alignment. And, of course, vitamins — those substances our bodies do not produce but which are nevertheless essential to normal brain function — must be present in adequate amounts. Usually the amount of vitamins necessary to produce the desired beneficial effects is relatively small.

Vitamins A, D, E, C, and all the B vitamins (including biotin) play important roles in maintaining our brain processes. It is certain of the B vitamins which, when lacking or deficient in our diets, can most easily produce a loss of vital memory. I focus on three of them here: vitamin B-1, or thiamine; B-3, niacin or nicotinic acid; and B-12. Each of these three can have a most profound effect on our vital memory functions, and in fact on many other functions of our central nervous systems. I also discuss vitamin B-6.

Choline is another compound that some investigators include among vitamins essential for memory. Choline is not technically a vitamin since it is partially synthesized in the body and is present in larger quantities than any of the true vitamins. It is a component of the acetylcholine molecule, the neurotransmitter that is a vital part of the memory circuits. Patients with Alzheimer's disease who have severe recent-memory loss tend to have reduced levels of acetylcholine in the inner part of their temporal lobes.

Researchers have tested the effects of increased choline intake in preventing symptoms of memory loss, both in those of us who are aging normally and also in Alzheimer's patients. Some studies have shown that large amounts of choline are helpful in certain kinds of memory function, but the evidence that increasing the amount of choline has any significant effect in improving the loss of recent memory in patients who do have Alzheimer's disease is less convincing.

If you want to try taking increased amounts of choline (something I do myself), I suggest you take it in a highly purified form called PhosChol, a brand name for concentrated lecithin. In my own case I've found it to be very helpful, and I believe that it produces a real improvement in memory rather than a placebo effect.

Food Sources of B Vitamins

How did primitive man survive and keep from being vitamin deficient when there were no supplemental vitamins around? The primary source of vitamin B-12 for ancient peoples was meat and other animal products. With us, through the action of bacteria, vitamin B-12 is present in beef, beef liver, eggs, flounder, herring, liverwurst, mackerel, milk, and milk products. With an adequate amount of animal products, including fish, in their diets, people won't develop vitamin B-12 deficiency unless their bodies lack what is known as the "intrinsic factor," a chemical discovered by two doctors at the Boston City Hospital, which is present in gastric juice and whose role is to allow vitamin B-12 to be absorbed into the blood stream. If there is a lack or deficiency of this intrinsic factor, vitamin B-12 won't get into the blood stream even if the vitamin is plentiful in the food that's digested.

Conversely, even when an adequate amount of the intrinsic factor is available, vitamin B-12 deficiency will occur if there is not enough of the vitamin in the diet. This is the case with strict vegetarians because vitamin B-12 does not occur in vegetables or fruits, unless they are mixed with bacterial products in some way.

Niacin (vitamin B-3) too is present in many meat products: beef liver, the white meat of chicken, halibut, peanuts, pork, salmon, swordfish, tuna, turkey, and veal, as well as in brewer's yeast and sunflower seeds. Thiamine (vitamin B-1) occurs in beef kidney, beef liver, and especially in brewer's yeast, in addition to whole wheat flour, wheat germ, whole grain products, dried navy beans, rice bran, raw brown rice, salmon steak, and soybeans.

The requirements for certain B vitamins, especially thiamine, are increased with greater caloric intake, and that is especially true of the greater caloric intake associated with drinking large amounts of alcohol or alcohol products. Pellagra, a disease occurring when niacin is deficient, is more common in countries that depend on maize or corn as a principal element in the diet.

People who don't have a deficiency of the intrinsic factor in their gastrointestinal mucosa, and whose diets are normal, including the substances we have enumerated, are unlikely to have a deficiency in these three B vitamins. However, persons on a reducing diet, or elderly people whose dietary intake is compromised by poor teeth or lack of appetite, may require supplementation.

The Major B Vitamins: Deficiency Syndromes Producing Memory Loss

Vitamin B-1 (Thiamine) Deficiency   Neurologists see many patients who are both alcohol abusers and victims of malnutrition. A number of them have persistent memory loss, even after they get massive vitamin therapy. Some neurologists got the idea that it might be possible to prevent some of the bad results of alcohol abuse by persuading the liquor, beer, and wine industries to add certain B vitamins to their beverages, and I went so far as to write a formal letter to one of the biggest distillers of alcohol, imploring the company to add thiamine to its product — an action that, if it were undertaken on a large scale, would save the useful lives of many thousands of people every year. Unhappily, the company's directors didn't think this was necessary.*

Today, alcohol producers go right on making their potent brain poisons, which are consumed by millions of Americans on a regular basis, without any thought as to how they can reduce the damage. In a way they're almost worse than cigarette manufacturers, who at least put filters on their cigarettes to try

*Federal regulations against adding vitamins directly to brain poisons such as alcoholic beverages could be overcome by attaching packages of B vitamin capsules to each bottle of alcoholic beverage.

to reduce the amount of tar and nicotine which is inhaled. But the liquor distilleries refuse to put thiamine in their products, or even package it separately and dispense it along with the beverages, which would help stop the memory loss associated with this deficiency.

Helene was a victim of the liquor industry who was caught in time. A sixty-two-year-old retired secretary living in a modern suburb with a small garden apartment and a failing marriage, she had blunted her emotional disappointment with an increasing daily ration of white wine, and subsequently vodka (vodka because she was under the impression that it did not leave a detectable odor on her breath). She would begin drinking early in the morning and often neglected to eat. On several occasions her husband had committed her to a mental hospital for the treatment of alcohol abuse, but when she came home she would start drinking and starving herself, just as she had before.

One morning Helene's cleaning lady found her confused and irrational, called the police ambulance, and had her taken to the local hospital. It was several days before the doctors there called in a neurologist. He found her to be confused and apathetic, and she was suffering from nystagmus, an unusual jiggling of the eyeballs when she tried to look from one side to the other. The neurologist also found that Helene had lost a substantial amount of recent memory. After his examination he sent her to one of the large hospitals, where I saw her.

I found Helene's loss of recent memory to be extensive and very disabling. What tipped me off to the true nature of her confusional state, however, was some of the answers she gave to my questions. At first I discounted them because I thought they simply reflected her confusion. But then it became obvious that her statements had fictional elements that confusion alone couldn't explain.

She told me, for example, that she had six children, although her husband had previously informed me that the couple was

149

childless. She told me that she and her husband lived in a grand mansion in one of the most fashionable suburbs of Chicago, Illinois, but I found that her garden apartment in a suburb of Boston was modest, and that she and her husband barely scraped by because of some of the reckless and unpredictable expenditures she incurred under the influence of alcohol.

These tall tales constitute a clinical symptom called confabulation, and together with her abnormal eye movement and the profound loss of recent memory, the diagnosis of Wernicke's Korsakoff's psychosis and thiamine deficiency was a certainty. This diagnosis was based on the history of inadequate food and vitamin intake that often occurs in patients who consume an excessive amount of alcohol. The clinical syndrome involving abnormal eye movement and the subsequent loss of recent memory are typical of Wernicke's disease. Unfortunately, most victims of this disease have suffered significant and irreversible damage to the inner parts of their thalamus and hypothalamus.

Two neurologists working at the Boston City Hospital and the Massachusetts General, Maurice Victor and Ray Adams, spent years examining patients with vitamin deficiency and alcoholism. They and other researchers indicated that the principal culprit resulting in the destruction of the patients' vital memories, particularly their recent-memory functions, was a lack of thiamine. The patients simply couldn't remember one fact or incident that exceeded their attention span. When the attention shifted, recent memory disappeared.

Although it is rare, some patients had a combined deficiency of vitamins B-5 (pantothenic acid) and B-6 (pyridoxine) as well as a thiamine (B1) deficiency. I suspected that this might have been the case with Helene, so I treated her with massive doses of all three B vitamins, both intravenously and by mouth. After a short while she was able to take other nutritious foods as well. The clinical result was favorable in Helene's case because there was a rapid resolution of most of her signs and symptoms, including a return of her vital memory, with only a modest loss of recent memory.

It was lucky for Helene that she was treated promptly. Most patients with persistent symptoms such as hers do not get their memory functions back, even when they're given an adequate course of treatment with the B vitamins, because lasting structural damage has taken place in the center of their brains which makes memory loss permanent. That's why it's so important to get the message across to wineries, beer manufacturers, and especially distilleries: if you're going to sell brain poisons like alcohol, at least put some B vitamins in them or attach them to the bottle to reduce the bad effects. Adding vitamins wouldn't prevent cirrhosis of the liver or its associated bleeding from the esophagus, but at least it would slow down brain deterioration.

Finally, I want to emphasize again that thiamine deficiency is in itself more important than alcohol abuse in causing memory loss. Severe thiamine deficiency, without alcohol abuse, has at times caused memory loss, although in our society such cases are unusual, and thiamine deficiency alone generally produces peripheral neuritis and numbness as its most outstanding features.

Additional thiamine in the diet can be very helpful, not only for alcoholics, but also for people who are drug dependent. A 1997 study by the department of psychiatry at the University of Connecticut emphasizes that point. The research project evaluated the effects of thiamine on memory task performance and event-related electroencephalographic (EEG) potentials in eight formerly cocaine-dependent patients. The patients orally ingested five grams of thiamine and/or five grams of a lactose placebo on two separate days, scheduled approximately one week apart. The order of administration was randomized, and double-blind procedures were followed. Approximately three hours after ingesting the capsules, patients completed a special memory scanning task and had event-related potentials on their EEGs simultaneously recorded. Thiamine was found to significantly improve recognition accuracy versus the placebo. Furthermore, the improvement was most reliable under conditions of increased memory load.

The results really shouldn't be too surprising, since the beneficial effects of adding thiamine to the diet were substantiated fifty years ago. That research, carried out in 1946 on eleven-year-old children in an orphanage, contradicted the prevailing medical view about nutrition and the amount of thiamine that is necessary in the diet. At the time, nutritionists felt that a maintenance level of thiamine in the diet was between 1.0 and 1.3 milligrams. The children who were being studied ate the same daily menus, which supplied about 1.0 milligram of thiamine a day. Over several years, a thiamine supplement was supplied in a scientifically controlled manner. The investigators found that those children who received the supplement, as opposed to the placebo, had significant improvement in intelligence, visual acuity, and memory. They also had a decrease in reaction times; that is, they were mentally quicker than the children who were given placebos. Today we know that 1.5 milligrams of thiamine is the absolute minimum daily required dose, and that 20.0 milligrams is an optimal dose.

Pellagra: Vitamin B-3 (Niacin) Deficiency   At one time state mental hospitals were inhabited by a lot of patients who were all classified as "crazy." The leading cause of their insanity was not schizophrenia or manic-depression; it was syphilis of the brain, an infectious disorder transmitted by a spirochete that produces a serious loss of many brain functions. The second leading cause was not an infection but a deficiency disease called pellagra, which tends to affect persons eating a diet consisting mostly of corn or maize since these foods do not supply enough niacin to meet the body's needs.

Today pellagra is unusual in the United States because many of the foods we buy in the supermarket, particularly most commercially baked breads, have added niacin. Pellagra is now largely restricted to underdeveloped countries, especially among the black population of South Africa.

I still remember my father, a general practitioner, showing me one of his patients, a farmer whom he treated in his practice back in the Great Depression. I was particularly struck by the man's lesions on areas of his skin exposed to sunlight.

This sick farmer had a couple of other important symptoms. He complained of abdominal cramps and diarrhea, and his wife said that he was depressed and didn't respond very well, and he kept forgetting what he had to do around the farm. One other thing worried her most of all. She turned to my father and said, "Do you think he's going mental?"

My father didn't then know that pellagra was a disease caused by a deficiency of niacin; when he saw this man, niacin hadn't yet been identified. He did know, however, that it was a deficiency disease, and he put the farmer on milk, yeast, and liver — foods he paid for out of his own pocket. The man's mental symptoms quickly disappeared.

Now, of course, we know that this disorder can be treated with niacin. Sometimes pyridoxine (vitamin B-6) is also needed to reverse the symptoms completely.

Vitamin B-6 and Folic Acid (Folate)   Vitamin B-6 (or pyridoxine) is a vitamin that has to be used very carefully because too much can cause a problem with sensation. However, we all certainly do need adequate amounts of it for good central nervous system function, both alone and in conjunction with other vitamins and minerals. For example, it has been shown that if we have insufficient levels of vitamin B-6 and folate, our plasma concentrations of the amino acid homocysteine may become elevated. This can increase the risks of blood vessel disease and the formation of blood clots in blood vessels, including those that supply the brain. In other words, therapeutic concentrations of vitamin B-6 and folate are likely to reduce the risk of heart attacks and strokes.

Folic acid is known to be extremely important for the normal development of the neural tube in the human embryo. We now have conclusive evidence that the incidence of neural tube defects and spina bifida can be reduced significantly if the amount of folic acid is increased in the diet of pregnant women. Thus, we should not be too surprised to find that folic acid supplements may yet prove to be helpful in the function of the mature central nervous system. Its relationship to vitamin B-12, as described below, tends to bear this out.

Vitamin B-12 Deficiency   A deficiency of vitamin B-12 can occur in the body even though an individual has an adequate diet. A special factor present in the gastric juice, the intrinsic factor, allows vitamin B-12 in our food to be absorbed into the blood stream. When this factor is missing, we can have a vitamin B-12 deficiency even though there's plenty of this vitamin in our food.

When vitamin B-12, along with folic acid, is deficient, a disease called pernicious anemia results. This condition is associated with combined degeneration of the spinal cord as well as a disease of the brain. The anemia can be cured with folic acid, but only vitamin B-12 can cure the diseases affecting the brain and spinal cord, which can produce numbness, spasticity and weakness of the muscles, signs of brain changes ranging from irritability to apathy and emotional instability, and finally a great loss of vital memory, with confusion or intellectual deterioration.

There are methods of measuring levels of vitamin B-12 in the blood. Classical nutritionists determined standards of what sufficient amounts of this vitamin were, without which an individual might get spinal cord disease or severe brain disease, including dementia and memory loss. Recent studies have shown, however, that the classical nutritionists set their standards too low, and that even when the amount of vitamin B-12 in the blood falls in the low-normal range, major neurobehavioral symptoms, including apathy, can occur.

Hildy was a twenty-three-year-old graduate student who was almost fanatical about avoiding any kind of poison — cigarettes, alcohol, or any sort of tainted food — and was also a strict vegetarian. She began to have symptoms of fatigue and memory loss, which were troublesome to her in her quite demanding studies. Eventually she came to see me, complaining of serious recent memory loss.

A complete evaluation disclosed that her vitamin B-12 level was in the low-normal range. She was not lacking the intrinsic factor, which promotes the absorption of vitamin B-12 into her blood stream; rather, Hildy was one of those vegetarians who just don't get enough vitamin B-12. I wasn't surprised at this because vegetarians, unless their food is contaminated by bacteria, have little if any of this vitamin in their diets. In Hildy's case, her vitamin B-12 level wasn't high enough to allow her brain to function normally. The addition of supplemental vitamin B-12 to her diet was enough to reverse her symptoms, disperse her depression, and improve her memory.

I'd like to stress this point to all vegetarians: if you're faithful to a regime of no meat or fish, you'll get very little if any vitamin B-12. This is an essential vitamin, and you must take vitamin supplements to maintain your nutritional balance. You may not feel in any way deficient or ill now, but once your body's store of vitamin B-12 is used up you'll run into precisely the same problems Hildy did. Moreover, people with pale blue eyes and a lack of hydrochloric acid in their stomachs are more likely than others to get pernicious anemia, a tendency that may be genetically determined. Such patients lack the intrinsic factor, and for them vitamin B-12 must be given by intramuscular injection — oral supplements are not effective.

A Balanced Diet and Vitamin Supplements

I'm often asked whether it's a good idea for those of us who eat a so-called balanced diet to take vitamin supplements, particularly of the B vitamins. In my opinion, because many of us eat less food as we grow older since we are less active and burn fewer calories, it is wise to add essential vitamins to make up for our reduced intake from the foods we eat.

I don't recommend megavitamin consumption because most of the excess vitamins are excreted in the urine and toxic concentrations of others can result. But based on what I've seen in my own medical practice, I believe that most people can benefit from taking larger amounts of vitamins — larger, that is, than the amounts recommended by classical nutritionists. I discuss in detail what I think are optimal levels of vitamins for various age groups in a subsequent chapter.

Finally, chemical tests of your blood can be carried out to determine whether or not you have an adequate concentration of B vitamins in your blood stream. Unless you have symptoms of Korsakoff's psychosis or beriberi, vitamin B-12 and folate are the vitamins usually tested for. These tests can be carried out by your doctor, and you may also consult with either your physician or a nutritionist to determine the proper dose of vitamin supplements you need. Most vitamin supplements contain extra vitamins that you may or may not need. There is a real danger of taking too much of certain vitamins, particularly the fat-soluble ones, which may have negative effects on your health. A doctor or nutritionist can help you avoid these complications. In addition, your doctor may prescribe extra vitamins if you are on any medicine that can deplete vitamin reserves, such as Dilantin, which uses up the body's store of vitamin D and, at times, certain B vitamins.

The routine laboratory tests we carry out on every patient who complains of memory loss include a hemogram with red blood cell indices to identify, for example, pernicious anemia, with associated folate and vitamin B-12 deficiencies. Most physicians conduct these examinations twice a year on their elderly patients, so a diagnosis of pernicious anemia is not likely to be missed. The isolated deficiency of vitamin B-12, however, is more likely to be undiagnosed, which is why we prescribe vitamin B-12 injections for our memory loss patients, even when their vitamin B-12 levels are in the low-normal range.

Vital Memory Points to Remember

1. As you get older and require fewer calories, you may need extra vitamins to replenish body stores.
2. Many elderly people don't get enough B vitamins.
3. A lack of vitamin B-1, B-3, or B-12 can readily produce a loss of vital memory.
4. Strict vegetarians *must* take supplements of vitamin B-12.

12

The Chemistry of the Body
and How It Affects the Mind
(Especially Vital Memory)

Electrolytes and the Brain

IF YOU'VE EVER BEEN with a very elderly or sick person when he or she became dehydrated, especially on a hot and humid day when fluid and electrolytes are lost through the lungs and skin and aren't replaced, you've noticed that the person began to have changes in mental functioning. One of the first problems encountered is a loss of memory. This happened to Muriel, one of my patients. Fortunately, I was there to observe the changes and reverse them with proper treatment.

Muriel, seventy-eight, a retired office administrator, was a slender, white-haired lady who was in the hospital to be treated with antibiotics for lung infection that interfered with her breathing. Massive doses of antibiotics had conquered the infection and she seemed to be on the road to recovery, but I was asked to examine her neurologically because one of her doctors thought she had a mental problem.

When I first saw her, about nine o'clock one morning, I carried out the routine tests, which showed her mental status functions — particularly her memory — to be normal. But because of the press of my schedule that day, I couldn't finish my examination, and I told her I'd be back after noon.

Muriel was in a two-bed hospital room without air conditioning. Mid-July in Boston can be hot, humid, and extremely uncomfortable. When I returned to examine her around 2:00 P.M., five hours later, I found that she had undergone a profound change in mental function, and her recent memory had declined to zero out of three.

At first I couldn't understand what might have produced this dramatic change in Muriel's mental abilities. Was her pneumonia worse, was she coughing, was she feverish, did she have trouble breathing? None of these was the answer.

What had happened was that Muriel was scheduled to have a special chest x ray, and through some miscommunication the nursing staff thought she was to have nothing by mouth before the exam. Over a long period of intense heat and humidity in the hospital room, Muriel received no fluids; in fact, she hadn't eaten or drunk anything since five o'clock the previous evening. A check of her blood electrolytes showed that her body water was depleted and that the concentration of sodium in her serum was extremely elevated.

Dehydration can actually produce shrinkage of the brain, and besides the kind of mental changes I found in Muriel, the patient may become very irritable. If she hadn't been treated promptly, she might have had even worse problems, including stupor. Because she was somewhat nauseated it was thought best to replace her deficient fluids intravenously. An IV infusion was done slowly because too rapid a correction of fluid imbalance can cause problems in other organ systems, and even in the brain itself.

The slow replacement of Muriel's fluids and electrolytes, giving her small amounts of potassium in a very dilute solution, brought her blood chemistry back to normal. Her depleted potassium rose, and her excessive sodium concentration slowly decreased to the normal range. Her nausea disappeared, and she was able to supplement the intravenous fluids by drinking appropriately buffered, not too distasteful liquid concoctions. Two days later she returned to her usual state of health and brain function and was discharged.

Most of us have had the experience of mental fatigue and slight memory problems, or even of feeling faint, while working or exercising in hot and humid weather. We have also been told on radio and television to drink extra fluids in such conditions and consume salt pills or drinks like Gatorade which contain potassium. If we don't replace fluids and electrolytes in a timely fashion, it should not surprise us that our symptoms will be severe.

In fact, confusion and even stupor may result when the concentration of various ions, or electrolytes, in the serum of the blood that irrigates the brain becomes unbalanced. When that imbalance affects the fluids surrounding the brain cells, and particularly the membranes of those brain cells, the most severe reactions occur, as happened to Muriel.

Although some neurologists find no evidence that memory itself is compromised in confusional states, when orientation to time, place, and even person is lacking, I contend that this state represents a severe loss of vital memory. The fact that the clinical syndromes associated with electrolyte imbalance may progress to stupor or even coma, on the one hand, or hyperirritability and epileptic seizures, on the other, indicates the importance of electrolyte concentrations, particularly across the membranes of nerve cells and brain fibers.

What Electrolytes and Ions Do

An electrolyte is a chemical that in a solution such as water, or especially blood, dissociates into ions. These ions have a small electric charge, either positive or negative, and are found both inside and outside the membranes of nerve cells and fibers. They help control the excitability of nerve elements and the conduction and propagation of electrical impulses in nerve fibers. The actual concentration of ions within and around nerve cells depends to some extent on the concentration of ions in the serum of the blood that circulates to and from the brain.

There are a number of important ions, such as sodium, potassium, chloride, calcium, magnesium, and carbonate, whose concentration can fluctuate only within a small range if the brain cells and brain mechanisms are to function properly. In a normal person, eating a nutritious diet and drinking sufficient but not excessive amounts of fluid ensure that the homeostatic regulation of ions and electrolytes is within normal limits. The acid-base balance is regulated in the same way, as described later in this chapter.

Probably the most important ion in the human body is the sodium ion. Its concentration in both the blood and the brain is related to the amount of water in and around the cells, particularly brain cells. When water becomes less plentiful, the concentration of sodium ion can increase dramatically, which may result in serious memory loss and rapid decline in mental abilities.

The reverse problem of too much water in the body can also occur, especially in hot weather when people perspire freely, losing salt in their perspiration and replacing it only with water or, as sometimes happens at sporting events, large amounts of beer. This overhydration can produce swelling of tissues and even of the brain. Again, not only vital memory but other aspects of mental function can be deranged. Drowsiness, giddiness, headaches, and nausea are quite common. Some people, especially those who are seizure-prone, may suffer convulsions if they become too waterlogged without taking in sufficient amounts of salt.

How do you tell whether major changes in electrolyte levels, and a loss of brain function possibly resulting in confusion, have occurred in elderly people, who may already be somewhat confused? They may have had memory loss or other symptoms that put them into the hospital or nursing home in the first place. The most important feature of diagnosis is a good history. In other words, establishing a neurological base line of the patient's function is critical so that one can determine if there is a change in personality, a worsening of intellectual abilities, or an increase in memory loss. If these things occur definitely and rather quickly, as happened with Muriel, a previous recent neurological evaluation will point that out. In her case, I was able to act quickly and decisively because I was certain that her neurological status indicated a change for the worse, and *blood tests* confirmed that she had an electrolyte and water imbalance.

Low Sodium Syndrome

One other note, on low serum sodium syndrome, which is just the reverse of Muriel's problem. This syndrome can occur in severely head-injured patients because of inappropriate hormonal secretion, particularly of the antidiuretic hormone from the posterior pituitary. Patients who have this problem excrete urine that is supersaturated with sodium, but they retain water and quickly develop low sodium levels in their blood and around their nerve cell membranes. This condition exacerbates their brain problems and makes them susceptible to confusion, coma, and epileptic seizures.

You mainly need to concern yourself with electrolyte levels if:

- you are elderly and subjected to long spells of hot weather
- you are on a special diet — for example, a low-salt diet — and live in an excessively warm environment
- you are taking medicines that may cause a change in your electrolyte levels (ask your doctor about this)
- you are chronically ill and are subjected to stressful circumstances

If you fall into one of these four categories, consult your doctor. Let your doctor treat you — don't try to treat yourself.

Ask for advice on the amount and kind of fluids which are right for you. If your doctor is in doubt, a simple blood test will determine whether or not you have an electrolyte imbalance. Your doctor can correct the imbalance by administering fluids or the electrolytes you are deficient in.

The Acid-Base Balance

The acid-base balance in and around the brain depends to some extent on the relationship between carbon dioxide and bicarbonate concentrations in the blood. Changes in the acid-base balance, for example in disease states such as diabetic coma, in which an increase in acidity occurs, affect brain function and memory. Acid-base imbalance is only one form of metabolic imbalance. A number of diverse disorders can produce such imbalances, and these disorders, which secondarily derange brain function, have their origin in the malfunction of other organ systems in the body, including the heart, lungs, kidney, liver, pancreas, and endocrine glands.

The acid-base imbalance is a relatively common metabolic disturbance that frequently causes brain dysfunction, or at least temporary deterioration in brain function, and loss of memory.

This imbalance is commonly experienced by people when they overbreathe when they're not actually working or running or exercising, and they blow off too much carbon dioxide as well as reduce the ionized calcium in their serum. They feel giddy and extremely dizzy. If one tests their mental status during this time there is a decrease in certain mental functions, including memory, as is illustrated in the case of Carrie, a thirty-seven-year-old mother of four.

One Saturday morning as she was pushing her shopping cart through the aisles of a supermarket, Carrie noticed that she was getting dizzy. If she hadn't had the shopping cart to lean on she would have fallen down. Moreover, she didn't know what items to select from the shelf. (She had never had this trouble before; her memory was good enough that she never used a shopping list.)

As Carrie became increasingly dizzy and confused she got a tingling sensation in her fingers, and she panicked. She ran out of the store and sat in her car for a long while until she gradually recovered. She was obviously disturbed by the mysterious ailment, but she didn't seek medical help until it happened again a short time after that. When it happened a third time she was referred to me to rule out some seizure disorder.

Carrie did not have seizures, and all her brain tests were normal. What she did have was a disturbance in her acid-base balance because she was hyperventilating and blowing off a large amount of carbon dioxide. The reason she was hyperventilating was that, because of problems with her husband, she was suddenly under a great deal of stress and in a state of emotional turmoil.

If you want to know how Carrie felt, all you have to do is breathe in and out rapidly and deeply for one to three minutes, and you'll begin to notice the same dizziness and fuzziness. Actually it's not necessary to overbreathe purposely to achieve this result. If you have a feeling of being trapped, you may begin to overbreathe quite unconsciously but with the same result.

The treatment of Carrie's acid-base problem was quite simple. All she had to do was to hold her breath. And if she couldn't do that she could hold a paper bag over her mouth so that she could rebreathe her own carbon dioxide. Dealing with the stress that made her overbreathe in the first place was the next thing she had to work on.

If you ever have an acid-base problem from overbreathing, you can quickly reverse the dizziness and fuzzy mental function by heeding the advice I gave to Carrie. Just stop breathing for a short while, or hold a paper bag over your mouth until the symptoms disappear.

Homeostasis and Memory

Although homeostatic mechanisms exist in the brain and although the pituitary and other endocrine glands secrete hormones to keep the water and electrolyte balance within a very narrow range of normal, dietary excess and dietary deficiency can change these concentrations, producing a decrease in many mental functions, including memory. Foods therefore must contain a sufficient amount of sodium, potassium, chloride, calcium, and magnesium, and intake of water should be adequate.

Normal concentration of water and electrolytes depends on proper excretion as well as adequate intake. In other words, a dysfunction or malfunction in the kidneys can cause a retention of waste products such as urea in the blood as well as an elevation of potassium. Routine chemical tests of your blood can determine whether you have this condition. If you have memory problems, make sure your doctor does these tests. Unfortunately for Laurence, his doctor did not do them in time.

Laurence was an eighty-two-year-old insurance salesman who had a probable case of Parkinson's disease, advancing rather slowly over a five- to six-year period. He was living in his own apartment with some occasional nursing assistance. Although he had problems orienting himself when he walked around the block, he was able to converse over the telephone and even talk knowledgeably about the stock exchange (and, incidentally, predict more accurately what was going to happen to the Dow Jones industrial average than some of the financial pundits seen on national television).

Laurence also had an enlarging prostate, which kept him from emptying his bladder. Over a period of time, urinary retention caused a dilatation of his ureters and finally a backup of urine into the kidneys themselves, which began to fail. Laurence didn't complain about his symptoms, and his doctor didn't pick up on his condition until he became comatose, his serum potassium level greatly elevated. He was rushed to the hospital, his bladder was emptied, and finally he had a prostate operation to relieve the obstruction. He did recover, but his mental function never returned to its previous level.

The brain of a person with Parkinson's disease is more fragile than that of a normal individual of the same age. It is a brain that withstands insult much less well than a normal brain. Laurence's doctor's failure to notice a medical problem superimposed on brain disease is not uncommon, but it reveals an attitude that must be changed in the medical profession.

Finally, Laurence's kidney deterioration might not have progressed as far as it did yet still could produce an increased level of circulating potassium which would affect brain function adversely. Even an increase in the blood urea nitrogen may be associated with a decrease in memory function and some deterioration in intellectual ability. That's why it's critical to make certain that the dangers of urinary obstruction are appreciated and that medical or surgical means are used to correct it promptly.

The Importance of Homeostasis

To recap, the state of equilibrium called homeostasis results from feedback from regulatory processes in the brain, pituitary, and other organs such as the kidneys. These processes control the concentration of sodium, potassium, chloride, calcium, carbonate, and phosphate in the blood and in and around brain cells within very narrow limits. They also regulate the amount of water in and around brain cells as well as in other parts of the body.

Homeostasis of water and electrolytes in and around brain cells is essential because any deviation above or below the normal concentrations may result in altered brain function, even in people who are otherwise normal. That this effect is more pronounced in cases of brain disease or injury is not only because the diseased brain is more susceptible to damage, but also because those homeostatic mechanisms originating in the brain may be deficient or absent. Maintaining water and electrolyte balance by adequate fluid and electrolyte administration in the elderly, particularly if they have symptoms of brain dysfunction, is essential.

The point I want to stress here is that homeostatic mechanisms may be more fragile in your elderly parent or relative, and they are more easily disrupted by disease states, particularly those affecting the brain. If the homeostatic mechanisms are fragile, your loved one must make a special effort to compensate. A person can do so by judicious intake of water and electrolytes, which is particularly important at times of stress — on very hot days, for example.

Even in completely healthy individuals like you and me, the body's homeostatic mechanisms can break down under conditions of extreme stress: when running a marathon, say, or crossing the Sahara, or climbing a peak in the Himalayas. Otherwise the mechanisms work well most of the time for people in good physical condition. The body is generally completely self-regulating, continually sending messages to the brain when it needs food, water, or oxygen. Homeostasis keeps the body chemistry at optimal levels of functioning all the time, until some extreme force or forces upset the balance. When that happens, it's usually wisest to seek immediate medical assistance.

If you faint on a hot day, or begin looking gray, or feel clammy and sick, ask your doctor to see you as an emergency patient in the office, or have your physician meet you at the emergency room of your local hospital. If you can't locate your doctor, the emergency room physician on duty is your best bet. If you or someone you know has collapsed, call an ambulance. The police or fire department will need to get you to the hospital for immediate treatment.

167

Vital Memory Points to Remember

1. An electrolyte is a chemical that, in solution, dissociates into ions. Sodium, potassium, chloride, calcium, magnesium, and carbonate are some of the important ions.
2. When someone in fragile health takes too much or too little water, a temporary electrolyte imbalance can occur which can cause memory loss.
3. The acid-base balance in the blood depends on carbon dioxide and bicarbonate concentrations.
4. Hyperventilation is the most common way that acid-base balance is disturbed.

13

Memory and Brain Metabolism

HAVE YOU EVER SEEN a very sick friend or relative with severe heart, lung, or liver disease — severe enough that the person had failing memory and intellect or delirium and stupor? And were you told that this deterioration was happening even though there was nothing intrinsically wrong with the person's brain? Such cases occur, not infrequently, illustrating that the brain does not work independently. Many organs of the body, especially the heart, which pumps blood to the brain, and other organs such as the liver, kidneys, lungs, and endocrine glands, must function adequately in order to support the activities of the brain. If you have a disorder of one of these organ systems and suffer failing memory or a loss of intellectual abilities, consult your physician for diagnosis and treatment because symptoms in this case often reflect a medical problem. Taking corrective actions on your own is apt to be counterproductive.

Blood Sugar and Vital Memory
Central to normal brain function are the life-giving nutrients: sugar, ketone bodies, and the oxygen necessary to metabolize them. Blood sugar levels are sensitive to ingested simple sugars so that it is possible, by eating large amounts of

169

simple sugars, to drive blood sugar up to very high levels, producing an excessive insulin response. For the most part, however, blood sugar level is the result of complex metabolic mechanisms.

Sugar in the blood results from the breakdown of a number of complex foods containing, among other things, large carbohydrate molecules such as starch as well as amino acids. The degradation of amino acid carbon skeletons occurs in the liver, which converts these skeletons to glucose. By a different metabolic route the carbon skeletons can be converted to fatty acids, or to what are known as ketone bodies. Glucose and ketone bodies can be directly metabolized in the brain, although ketone bodies are also metabolized by muscles.

The brain's major fuel in a nonstarving human being on a mixed diet is glucose. In starvation states, ketone bodies are also used as fuel by the brain.

You don't need to understand the complexities of how sugars are metabolized, or what the body uses for fuel, but you should know that the concentration of sugar in the blood is normally kept within certain finite limits. If it's too high, as in diabetes mellitus, where insulin is insufficient, sugar and ketone bodies are spilled into the urine and the acid-base balance in the blood is disturbed. Severe acidosis then occurs which, if it persists, will result in diabetic coma.

Of course, vital memory is destroyed by any condition that can cause coma. The treatment for diabetes involves both an adequate amount of sugar and the right dosage of insulin. Since the treatment of patients in diabetic coma is usually handled by an internist and not a surgeon, I wasn't thinking about the treatment of diabetic coma when I went to sleep one night in the interns' quarters at the University of Minnesota Hospital.

I had been on duty for thirty-six continuous hours, most of which I spent in the operating room. The intern who had the bed next to mine (his last name also began with an *M*) was on the internal medicine rotation, in the service specializing in treating patients with diabetic coma.

I had only been asleep for fifteen or twenty minutes when the telephone rang, and my first thought as I answered the phone was that some emergency must have come up in one of my surgical cases. The head nurse I talked with said that the patient (I couldn't get the name) was in a diabetic coma, and I proceeded to give her instructions about the amounts of insulin and glucose needed to treat the patient. She called me about every thirty to thirty-five minutes during the rest of the night. As soon as I finished each conversation with her I would go back to sleep, only to have the telephone awaken me with another request for instructions.

I was more than a little baffled the next morning when my medical neighbor, the doctor whose last name also began with the letter *M*, thanked me profusely. "Gee," he said, "you did a beautiful job of treating my patient with diabetic coma. She's alert and bright as a penny now." I was astonished, since I had very little recollection of what had gone on during the night. But I confirmed that the telephone calls hadn't been about my patient at all, and that I had inadvertently treated a patient I had never seen or heard of before.

Of course, I went to see the twenty-six-year-old patient the next morning. The onset of her coma had been associated with fatigue, weakness, and abdominal pain as well as headache. She then became confused, with disorientation and a loss of vital memory functions before she went into stupor, and was brought into the University Hospital with Kussmaul breathing, a peculiar kind of breathing characteristic of patients in diabetic coma. When I saw her she still seemed fatigued and weak, but her confusion had disappeared and her vital memory had returned to the extent that she knew where she was and what was happening to her.

The lesson to be drawn here is that persons with diabetes who are having memory or mental difficulties should consult their physicians immediately for testing and corrective treatment because these symptoms often indicate a medical problem.

Low Blood Sugar

I'm sure that at some point you have "pigged out" on candy, ice cream, or rich desserts, only to find a couple of hours later that you felt fatigued and even tremulous. You may have suffered an insulin rebound effect from taking too much sugar, which results not in high blood sugar but just the opposite — low blood sugar, or hypoglycemia.

A severe form of this syndrome occurs in people with insulin-secreting tumors of the pancreas, but low blood sugar is also seen in those facing intense stress who are also insulin hypersecreters. In one study a series of medical students had their blood sugar levels taken before and then two hours into an important examination. A surprising number of them had depressed blood sugars. In other words, at a time when they needed their mental resources most, many of them felt weak, tremulous, and had abdominal pain — not a good combination for the best results on an exam.

Harry was a thirty-six-year-old medical student who had such symptoms; glucose tolerance tests showed that his blood sugar went down to very low levels. He went to get a physical examination when he found that his performance was deteriorating and his ability to remember key facts in the clinical cases he was handling had fallen to unacceptable levels.

A test for tumor of the pancreas luckily came back negative. His physician, a gastroenterologist (that is, a doctor specializing in treating diseases of the gastrointestinal tract), decided to give him special medications. He also thought he would try a change in Harry's diet.

First, Harry was taken off all simple sugars: no more sweet

desserts, ice cream, or candy. His sources of carbohydrate were limited to starchy foods such as cereals, vegetables, potatoes, and bread. He was allowed to eat a fair amount of protein, especially chicken, turkey, and fish, and he had small meals more frequently dispersed during the day. One of the snacks he enjoyed was peanut butter. Peanut oil contains a substantial amount of monounsaturated fatty acids, a relatively harmless kind of fat. This fat did two things to aid Harry's problem: first, it slowed the emptying of his stomach, and second, it made the supply of nutrients in Harry's blood, and in turn to his brain, more evenly distributed, so that an excessive amount of insulin was not secreted.

It is important to recognize and treat hypoglycemia because, in its extreme form, it can cause not only confusion but also epileptic convulsions, postconvulsion stupor, and finally a prolonged state of unconsciousness. If the blood sugar goes down to 30 mg per 100 cc's, confusion, disorientation, and loss of vital memory are all very severe, and it is at this point that epileptic seizures may occur. If the blood sugar goes down to 10 mg per 100 cc's, a profound loss of consciousness results which may produce irreversible damage to the brain. Fortunately, most of us who suffer low levels of blood sugar don't have these severe problems or display such alarming symptoms. We may become nauseated and somewhat tremulous and apprehensive, and our abilities to do complicated intellectual functions, including those that require good recent memory for new learning, are impaired.

If you suspect you have any of these symptoms, see your doctor because the implications of low blood glucose can be verified or disproved by blood tests. Blood sugar levels can be taken after fasting, then a measured amount of glucose is usually taken by mouth and blood sugar tests repeated at 30, 60, 90, 120, 180, and occasionally 240 minutes. Insulin levels can also be determined. If these tests are abnormal, you should seek the attention of a doctor who specializes in blood sugar problems to determine the precise cause. For most people an imbalance in blood sugar is minor and not life-threatening, and the symptoms can often be completely eradicated by changing the diet, as in Harry's case.

Oxygen and Memory Loss

The reduced oxygen supply to the brain in persons with severe anemia or heart or lung disease can cause memory loss. Brain cells, of course, need oxygen. A constant supply of oxygen depends on normal functioning of the heart, and a heart that is failing may not be able to pump blood at the proper rate to supply nutrients and oxygen to the brain. Also, if the blood vessels to the brain are partially occluded or clogged by arteriosclerosis, the amount of blood and therefore oxygen reaching the brain may be insufficient. But even if the heart is working perfectly and the blood vessels are clear, oxygen may be diminished because of lung disease in which too little oxygen is exchanged at the lung capillaries and thus not enough is supplied to support normal function of brain cells. When the lungs are working normally and enough oxygen is delivered into the blood, the oxygen must still be picked up by the hemoglobin, a blood compound containing iron, in the red blood cells. Lack of iron can produce iron deficiency anemia, which can be so severe that an insufficient amount of oxygen is carried to the brain.

Timothy was a forty-three-year-old iron worker who had suffered a head injury at work. He wasn't knocked unconscious and didn't lose his memory when he was injured, but afterward he had great difficulty carrying out his normal functions, was easily fatigued, and couldn't think. His memory abilities, particularly his vital memory functions, were impaired. Timothy's doctors thought that his symptoms were related to his head injury. But when I reviewed his case, more than five years after his accident, it didn't seem to me that Timothy's disabilities all stemmed from a trivial head injury.

I came to this conclusion when I looked over his medical chart in detail, including records dating from before the injury. At one time he had gone to a doctor claiming to be lightheaded, easily fatigued, and lacking in energy — the same complaints he had after the injury. He had even had a neuropsychological examination, one that was difficult to interpret. His mental functions, and particularly his memory functions, had deteriorated greatly after several hours of testing. The thing no one seemed to pick up on was his severe iron deficiency anemia, a problem that explained both his present symptoms and the abnormalities on his earlier neuropsychological tests.

The lowest limit of the normal range for serum iron is 50. Timothy's was 5, and his hemoglobin was also very low. No wonder he felt lightheaded and weak and fatigued easily No wonder he had memory failure and failure of mental function. The repeated blood studies, in spite of the fact that he was given supplemental iron, never came back to normal. It was my opinion that a lack of oxygen going to his brain had caused his mental problems. The heme component of the hemoglobin molecule lacked enough iron to hook the oxygen on to.

Timothy was trying to get a sizable settlement for his head injury from an insurance company, but I recommended that before any settlement was made he receive much more adequate treatment for his anemia. This wasn't as easy as it sounds. An iron-rich diet did not bring his serum iron level back to normal, and an extensive series of medical examinations revealed no reason for an extraordinary loss of iron (as, for example, through blood in the stools). Finally, when large amounts of supplementary iron were given, Timothy's serum iron gratifyingly increased to within the normal range, improving his ability to resist fatigue and somewhat restoring his memory and intellectual functions as well.

Some writers in the field of memory preservation and

memory loss do not believe that iron deficiency anemia can affect memory or other brain functions. However, a 1995 study carried out in Indonesia contradicts that point of view and supports my clinical impression.

The study investigated the relationship between iron deficiency and intellectual function, and the impact of iron supplementation on verbal intelligence, attention, and concept learning. One hundred seventy-six iron-deficient children were studied, some of whom had no anemia and some of whom were anemic. Half of the children, aged three to six years, received elemental iron for eight weeks, and the other half received a placebo. The study found that there were significant changes from before to after the intervention in the blood of the previously anemic children. Psychological tests carried out before and after treatment showed that iron deficiency anemia produced alterations in intellectual processes related to visual attention and concept acquisition. These alterations, related to memory, were reversed after treatment.

Another study assessed the impact of iron supplementation on infants with iron deficiency anemia. One hundred twenty-six anemic babies, ages twelve to eighteen months, were randomly assigned to receive either iron treatment or a placebo. After four months of iron supplementation, there was a striking improvement in the anemia. Also, the infants whose neurological development was significantly retarded before the iron treatment had normal neurological development when the anemia was reversed.

It is my impression that severe iron deficiency anemia seriously interferes with a person's ability to focus attention and concentrate. These abilities are vital for the proper encoding of memory. The increasing fatigue that often accompanies severe iron deficiency anemia further decreases these abilities, and further interferes with the memory process.

Of course, oxygen in the blood can also be decreased by any

kind of lung disease, such as pneumonia, chronic obstructive lung disease, and lung cancer — diseases often associated with cigarette smoking. Even continual cigarette smoking without obvious lung disease can reduce the amount of oxygen in the blood because of gases inhaled in the cigarette smoke, including carbon gases. It is not surprising, then, when a chronic smoker with lung infection and a smoker's cough exhibits lips and fingernails that are blue or cyanotic and is unable to carry out simple mental tasks because not enough oxygen is going to his brain cells.

Infections that result in a backup of fluids into the lungs — pneumonia, bronchitis, and disorders such as emphysema and congestive heart failure — can interfere with the exchange of oxygen, including the oxygenation of the blood running through the lung capillaries. There is very little that persons with this problem can do to help themselves. Deep breathing, for example, only causes carbon dioxide to be blown off, thereby producing dizziness.

Raising the amount of oxygen in inspired air increases oxygen concentration in the lung capillaries and thus the amount of oxygen going to the brain. But doing so means that an individual must be in an oxygen tent or have a nasal catheter in place through which a continuous flow of oxygen gas is bubbling.

The important factor with lung disease or bronchial tube infections is proper treatment. Sometimes what is required is antibiotic therapy to rid the lungs of infection. At other times the ability of the lungs and bronchial tubes to eliminate secretions that partially or completely plug parts of the respiratory system must be improved. Sometimes surgical treatment is necessary.

The combination of iron deficiency anemia and lung disease may reduce the oxygen level in the brain more sharply than either disease alone, and it is more apt to produce symptoms of reduced memory and mental ability than either disease alone. Of course, both conditions, the lung disease and the anemia, must be treated effectively to reverse memory loss and mental symptoms.

Prevention of Lung Disease

An even more important principle is that of lung disease prevention. Such prevention can be effected by improved working conditions for those involved in some aspects of mining, cotton processing, and other work that can damage the lungs. Avoiding active or passive cigarette smoke is also extremely important. Moreover, asthma must be treated promptly whenever it occurs so that the consequences of chronic lung disease can be avoided, and infections of the pharynx and nasopharynx which might spread into the lower respiratory system must be treated.

In my previous book, *Brain Power*, I gave the example of my old barber who had a smoker's cough and blue fingernails. He kept cutting the hair on one side of my head again and again, ignoring the side left uncut. It's not only barbers who have such problems. I've seen trial lawyers who were heavy smokers sitting in the same kind of dazed condition. And yes, I've even seen physicians with this problem.

An Overview

Vital memory and proper brain function depend on a normal supply of oxygen and glucose being delivered to brain cells through the arteries going to the brain. If the brain is deprived of oxygen for more than a few minutes at normal temperature, irreversible changes can occur in the inner parts of the temporal lobes. In other words, brain cells in the hippocampus, an area that is related to the laying down of new memories, may die.

Similarly, prolonged and deep hypoglycemia, that is, a severely depressed level of blood sugar, may result in convulsions. (Many years ago severe mental illness was treated by artificially producing convulsions through the injection of insulin, which brought about proportionally low levels of blood sugar.) Again, such convulsions cause scarring in the depths of the brain, including the hippocampus, and often resulted in a loss of vital memory.

Most problems related to a lack of sugar or of oxygen going to the brain can be readily treated and reversed. The important thing is to recognize the problem, find its source, and correct it promptly. Correction can mean changing one's diet, having lung problems treated, completely avoiding cigarette smoke, or having severe anemia treated. Whatever treatment measures are necessary, they usually produce a dramatic improvement, including an improvement in memory and brain function, in a relatively short time.

Vital Memory Points to Remember

1. The brain's major fuel is glucose, which must be supplied within certain finite limits for optimal brain and memory functions.
2. Extreme forms of hypoglycemia can cause confusion and epileptic convulsions.
3. Anemia can cause a loss of mental function and vital memory.
4. Cigarette smoking is the most common cause of low oxygen levels in the blood.

14

Thyroid Dysfunction and Memory Loss

WHAT DO YOU THINK of when someone talks about hormones? You most likely don't think of memory loss. Indeed, when the body's hormones are in proper balance there's no danger of their producing memory loss. But if they're out of kilter they can alter the brain's metabolism and chemical environment, which in turn can change brain function for the worse.

Hormonal Balance
You should understand something about hormonal imbalance because these abnormalities can be treated and reversed. Before I describe how hormonal imbalance can produce memory loss, however, you may need a little background on how hormones work and why they're important. Briefly, the brain is extremely dependent on the other organ systems of the body in order to function properly. Hormones secreted by the endocrine glands play an essential role in the process of maintaining homeostasis — keeping the brain's environment balanced.

The master gland that controls many hormones in the body is the pituitary, which is situated at the base of the skull in a little hollow of bone called the Turkish saddle. It is intimately connected with the hypothalamus, which controls fight-or-flight behavior, proper water balance, body temperature, and natural sleep patterns.

In conjunction with the pineal gland, these tissues regulate the rhythms of the body — not only the wake-sleep cycles but also such patterns as the daily and hourly variations in electrolytes, alterations in the level of clotting factors in the blood, changes in body temperature, and even some emotional changes. These hourly biological changes are called circadian rhythms.

Through various feedback mechanisms, the pituitary also controls the hormonal secretions of other endocrine glands throughout the body. These include the cortex of the adrenal gland, which secretes the steroid hormones; the islands of Langerhans in the pancreas, which secrete insulin (essential for the metabolism of sugar); the parathyroid glands, which control the concentration of calcium in the blood; and the thyroid gland, which controls the rate of metabolism in the body. The pituitary also controls the male testes, which secrete testosterone, and the female ovaries, which secrete estrogen compounds and progesterone.

Each of these hormones has an effect on brain function and memory, but one of the most common hormonal problems (aside from insulin–blood sugar variations) is brought on by decreased levels of thyroid hormone. While small deviations from the normal concentration of thyroid hormone can produce mild changes in brain function, severe memory loss is seen in full-blown cases of hypothyroidism.

Hypothyroidism

One afternoon late in 1989, after I had completed rounds with the neurology residents at a large urban hospital, one of them took me aside and asked me if I wanted to see Oscar, the residents' latest prize patient. He confided that they had just rescued Oscar, a fifty-six-year-old insurance underwriter, from one of the general medical services, which saw him as only another degenerate alcoholic. (The medical service had asked for a neurological consultation since the toxic screen was normal and there was no history of alcoholism.)

Oscar had looked like an alcoholic in almost every way. He was disheveled and hadn't shaved or bathed in a long time. He was sluggish in his movements and spent a lot of time just staring at the wall. He wasn't able to give a good account of himself because his memory processes were so slowed.

Blood studies showed that Oscar had severe hypothyroidism — that is, a lack of thyroid hormone secretions. When I saw him he had been cleaned and shaved and had already started treatment with thyroid hormone, but his mental processes were still extremely sluggish. Recent-memory testing showed that he could not remember any of three unrelated objects after a period of two and a half to three minutes, and his recollection of the weeks and months preceding his hospitalization proved to be incomplete and inaccurate. But I was certain his memory problems were reversible, and indeed, with persistent and effective treatment Oscar returned to normal health. A more accurate history taken once he had recovered indicated that he was not, in fact, an alcoholic. It's important to keep in mind, however, that the clinical picture produced by hypothyroidism is easy to misdiagnose as alcoholism, depression, or even Alzheimer's disease, particularly among the elderly, whose physicians often tell the patients' relatives that their gradual mental failure is to be expected — "There's nothing to do about it, it's just old age."

I've seen people similar to Oscar who had been misdiagnosed for many months in nursing homes. One such person benefited from a lecture my colleague, Tom Sabin, gave to a group of nursing home doctors. A doctor who heard Tom's lecture decided he'd test out some of his alleged Alzheimer's patients, and sure enough he found one who was suffering instead from hypothyroidism. The misdiagnosed man responded remarkably well to thyroid hormone. Within several months he had left the nursing home and moved to a rest home, where he was able to take complete charge of his daily activities — dressing, feeding himself, setting his own schedule, and even going out by himself.

Hyperthyroidism Leading to Hypothyroidism

The first case of hypothyroidism, mental deterioration, and memory loss I saw as an intern in 1947 resulted from surgical treatment rather than spontaneous disease causing destruction or malfunction of the thyroid gland. The patient was a forty-seven-year-old bakery clerk named Gloria, who initially had a severe case of hyperthyroidism, characterized by bulging eyes, agitation, irritability, and apprehension. She sometimes became manic and talked a blue streak, interrupted by sudden mood swings and weeping.

In treating her hyperthyroidism, Gloria's surgeon had removed so much of her thyroid gland that what remained did not produce an adequate amount of thyroid hormone. She went from being hyper-irritable to being dull, listless, and drowsy. Her speech became somewhat slurred, and her intellectual processes deteriorated because her memory functions were so slowed. She couldn't concentrate, and thus no new memories were acquired, and she had difficulty retrieving old memories from her memory bank. In other words, her thyroid surgery had transformed her from hyperthyroidism to profound hypothyroidism.

I'd like to be able to tell you that the cause of Gloria's problem was immediately understood since it was of course known that she had had much of her thyroid removed. But forty-five years ago this didn't happen, and she became demented before the true nature of her problem was discovered and she was put on thyroid hormone. Even so, treatment did finally reverse her abnormal mental syndrome.

Hypothyroidism can occur without a large portion of the

thyroid gland having been surgically removed. Ken, an eighty-two-year-old retired bank examiner, had a nodule removed from his thyroid which left most of the gland intact. He seemed to be functioning normally and went for his regular exercise, followed by a steam bath. He couldn't tolerate the steam, however, and he fainted. When he recovered consciousness he wasn't able to function at his previous level, and his doctor thought that he either had had a stroke or was getting Alzheimer's disease, with apathy and memory loss.

Ken subsequently developed an intestinal obstruction, and when he went into a hospital to have this problem surgically corrected it was discovered that his thyroid was underactive. Treatment with thyroid hormone restored him, even at age eighty-two, to normal mental activity. The moral to this story is that anyone who has had thyroid surgery or thyroid dysfunction in the past should have repeated tests of thyroid function to detect and treat abnormalities early so that the difficulties Ken and Gloria encountered can be avoided.

No one should be diagnosed as having Alzheimer's disease before a complete blood and urine evaluation is made by appropriate laboratory studies. Chemical analysis of the blood should always include a thorough check of thyroid function as well as measures of the effectiveness of the liver, the kidneys, and the other endocrine glands as well. Today the dementia and memory loss produced by abnormalities of the thyroid, adrenal cortex, insulin-secreting glands in the pancreas, parathyroid, and pituitary are too easy to diagnose and treat to allow any of them to cause memory loss and mental deterioration.

This is especially true of the hypersecretion of insulin, which depresses the blood sugar, whether the hypersecretion is caused by a pancreatic tumor, emotional lability, or excessive intake of sugar with an insulin rebound. Low blood sugar can readily be identified by blood tests, and treatment may involve only an adjustment in the diet to reverse memory impairment.

Different hormones related to the adrenal cortex may have quite different effects on memory. For example, stress- and treatment-induced elevations of the steroid hormone cortisol have been associated with impaired memory in otherwise healthy adults. An investigation carried out in Germany on thirteen subjects found that when they were exposed to a brief psycho-social laboratory stress, those subjects who responded with a high cortisol level had significantly poorer memory performance.

In a subsequent study, forty healthy subjects received either 10 milligrams of cortisol or a placebo. One hour later they were given memory tests. Subjects who received cortisol showed impaired performance in spatial thinking, but not in other memory tasks.

Some individuals who are hyper-reactors to stress may have chronically elevated cortisol levels in their plasma. It has been suggested that such an elevated level may be associated with structural changes in the hippocampus, the structure in the temporal lobe closely associated with the memory function. A study was carried out at Yale medical school using magnetic resonance imaging (MRI) to measure the volume of the hippocampus in twenty-six veterans with combat-related post-traumatic stress disorder. The results were compared to measurements taken of the volume of the hippocampus in normal controls; twenty-two comparison subjects, selected to be similar to the veterans in age, sex, race, years of education, socioeconomic status, body size, and years of alcohol abuse, had similar measurements taken of their hippocampus. Comparison studies showed that the post-traumatic stress disorder patients had a statistically significant decrease in the size of their right hippocampus as compared to the control subjects. In addition, they had deficits in their short-term verbal memory as measured by the Wechsler memory scale.

Pavlovian-like conditioning in some people who are hyper-reactors to stress has shown that they had decreases in their cortisol levels. This indicates, at least theoretically, that memory problems associated with increased cortisol levels may be treatable and reversible.

In humans of both sexes, dehydroepiandrosterone sulfate (DHEAS), an adrenally secreted steroid, circulates in blood but its serum concentration decreases with age. By the time people get to be eighty or ninety, the concentration of this steroid in the blood is only about 10 to 20 percent of its value in young adulthood. Whether there is a cause-and-effect relationship between the decreasing levels of this hormone with age and the physiological and pathological manifestations of aging is still undetermined. However, some investigators feel that the reduction in this hormone with aging may have significant neuropsychiatric effects.

For example, one study in California was carried out on six middle-aged and elderly patients with major depression and low plasma levels of this hormone. Significant amounts of the hormone (30 to 90 milligrams per day for four weeks) were given to them therapeutically in doses sufficient to achieve circulating plasma levels found in young healthy adults. All of these patients had significant improvements in their depression, and substantial recovery of memory performance.

A similar study was carried out in Germany in 1997. Forty healthy elderly men and women (mean age sixty-nine years) participated in a double-blind, placebo-controlled DHEAS substitution study. For two weeks subjects took 50 milligrams of DHEAS daily, followed by a two-week wash-out period and then followed by two weeks of placebo administration. The treatment sequence was randomized in a crossover design. Every two weeks, neuropsychological tests were administered.

In the beginning all subjects had low DHEAS baseline levels. However, the administration of the hormone produced substantial and measurable changes in blood studies, with a return to youthful levels. Unfortunately, the study did not show a concomitant strong beneficial effect of the hormone administration (with its elevation of the hormone level in the plasma), and the subjects did not have an improvement in their intellectual or memory abilities.

Research on the therapeutic effects of various adrenal hormones on memory function is, therefore, inconclusive. Nevertheless, drug stores and natural food stores sell these products without a prescription. Furthermore, some of these hormonal products may affect other bodily systems, such as the immune system, in ways that we cannot predict. The unknown effects of these hormones do not mean that certain kinds of hormone therapy will not have a therapeutic effect on brain function and memory. What it means is that we need better information on this subject. Clearly, more scientific research is indicated.

Brain functions and especially memory are very susceptible to changes in hormonal levels. And, of course, memory loss always impairs new learning. As a corollary, I believe that people with learning problems should have medical evaluations, including blood tests, to gauge hormonal levels accurately.

Vital Memory Points to Remember
1. Hypothyroidism (a lack of thyroid hormone) can produce clinical symptoms resembling those of alcoholism or even Alzheimer's disease.
2. Hyperthyroidism (too much thyroid hormone) can cause a range of symptoms, including a lack of concentration and hyperdistractibility with secondary memory loss.

PART IV

Diseases and Injuries That Cause Memory Loss

WHAT IMAGES are conjured up in your mind when you hear of people who have something wrong with their brains? Do you envision a person who acts crazy or stupid, someone who is losing intellectual capacity, or is unable to function, an individual who is comatose or delirious?

Certainly severe problems can afflict the brain, with very undesirable consequences. But remember also that brain sciences have made fantastic progress in the last three decades, in both the diagnosis and treatment of brain diseases and injuries. When pinpointed early, the causes of brain symptoms, especially memory loss, can in many cases be reversed. This fact is important for you to know because many people, when faced with the symptoms of memory loss, become quite depressed. Their first thought is that, like their fathers or grandmothers before them, they've got Alzheimer's disease, that everything is lost, and that there's nothing that can be done for them. Fortunately, that's not true in the vast majority of cases.

After you've read about the various problems described in Part IV you'll begin to see that many different conditions can cause memory loss, that many of them are treatable, and that memory loss is often reversible. It's also good to keep in mind that even people with degenerative brain disease, such as Alzheimer's disease, may have other disorders (like depression, brain poisoning with various drugs or alcohol, malnutrition, or electrolyte imbalance) superimposed on their problem, which make the memory loss much worse than it needs to be. Especially in the beginning stages of Alzheimer's, the prevention of or treatment of depression, brain poisoning, malnutrition, or some of the other problems detailed in this part can improve patients' clinical condition and reverse much of their memory loss.

We don't yet have a cure for Alzheimer's, but I do think it's important never to give up hope. Medical research is now being focused on the problems of degenerative brain disease, and they are soluble. It's simply a matter of time and money being applied to research that will ultimately discover the prevention and cure of these diseases. In the meantime, we must give the victims of Alzheimer's and other degenerative brain diseases the best possible treatment. The fewer medical complications they have, the longer they'll be able to live active, full, and interesting lives.

15

Brain Infections That Cause Memory Loss

WHEN WE CONSIDER brain infections that cause memory loss, we're looking at a chapter in medical history which has achieved some amazing triumphs. Many brain infections are completely treatable and curable, and there is hope that rapid progress will be made in conquering those infections, like AIDS, that are not curable at the present time.

Seventy years ago one of the leading causes of memory loss dementia and, indeed, insanity was syphilis of the brain. Now the overwhelming majority of patients with this affliction can be cured by massive doses of penicillin. Newer antibiotics can even cure some brain abscesses that previously had to be drained surgically. Infections caused by bacteria are most readily treated with antibiotics. But even some viral infections can be controlled by antiviral medications if they are given in time. This proved to be true in the case of Hector, a fifty-three-year-old plumber from Boston.

One Sunday several years ago I was called in to a local hospital to do a brain biopsy on Hector, who had a progressive infection of his brain with bizarre changes in personality and severe distortions in memory. Special tests of the brain showed swelling of both temporal lobes, and tests of the blood and spinal fluid gave evidence of infection. As Hector became more and more ill he had spells of delirium. A tentative diagnosis was made of herpes infection of the brain, so-called herpes encephalitis. This viral encephalitis tends to produce swelling of the temporal lobes and is associated with sudden, rapid changes in personality and severe distortions in brain function, including memory.

An experimental drug was then available which was at least partially effective in arresting herpes infection, but it was also quite toxic. Rather than give a drug that might prove to be inappropriate if the diagnosis was wrong and was in any case potentially lethal, brain biopsies were routinely required before the drug's administration so that the tissue could be cultured and a positive diagnosis of herpes infection of the brain confirmed.

Once the biopsy of Hector's brain had been done, the doctors who supervised the making of viral cultures expected to have a positive culture within twenty-four hours, and certainly within forty-eight. After two days had passed and the culture was still negative, they realized they might not be dealing with a herpes infection of the brain at all, but rather with a disease called Jacob Creutzfeldt's syndrome. This dreaded but extremely rare disease produces a rapid onset of dementia and loss of brain function. Absolutely no treatment for it exists. The peculiar organism, the prion, that causes the disease is very resistant to the usual methods of sterilization, and one of the few agents that is effective in sterilizing surgical instruments — that is, that will kill the organism — is chlorine bleach in concentrated solution. The suspicion that Hector's symptoms indicated Jacob Creutzfeldt's syndrome put the scrub nurses who had assisted with the biopsy in a panic because the sterile gloves they had worn had holes in them, and moreover one of them had a wound on her hand and was convinced that this fearsome organism had entered her body.

Finally, after ninety-six hours had passed, a positive diagnosis of herpes encephalitis was confirmed by Hector's culture, and the panic in the nursing staff abated. In the meantime, however, all surgical instruments were soaked in bleach solution, with the unhappy outcome of destroying some of the more delicate ones. The Jacob Creutzfeldt's scare in the operating room cost the hospital around $3,500 to replace these instruments. But Hector's case ended better: the new drugs against herpes encephalitis were effective, and Hector made a nice recovery, reverting to his normal personality and improved recent-memory function.

Brain infections can be caused by bacteria, fungi, protozoans, or viruses. They may be generalized in the brain, producing a disease like sleeping sickness, or they can be localized in one part of the brain. If the local infection is walled off by reactive tissue, it will form an abscess and has to be treated surgically by drainage or removal. Infections can invade the brain from infected nasal sinuses or mastoids or from infections in the blood. No matter how it occurs, any infection of the brain is a serious medical problem.

Infections of the entire brain, such as in encephalitis, may be closely related to infections of the tissues covering the brain, the meninges. These infections, called meningitis, are often characterized by high fever, headaches, and a stiff neck. If the meningeal infection spreads to the brain tissue, it may irritate brain cells enough to cause epileptic seizures. A correct diagnosis in cases of this kind is extremely important. If meningitis is suspected, a careful spinal puncture should be carried out to analyze the spinal fluid. With infants and young children especially, high fever alone, without any infection of the brain or spinal fluid, can trigger an epileptic convulsion in patients whose threshold for epileptic seizures is decreased.

Identifying Brain Infections

Many kinds of brain infection produce changes in personality and decrease memory abilities, including infections that are secondary to such viral diseases as measles. Some viral infections — herpes for instance — tend to localize in structures related to memory function, like the temporal lobes. This localization also occurs with the virus that causes rabies, which produces characteristic changes in the hippocampus as well as the most severe changes in personality and behavior. Its very name — in French, *rage;* in Italian, *rabia;* and in German, *Wut* — means "madness" or "rage."

The recognition of acute brain infections is usually not difficult. The patient becomes very ill with fever, and noticeable changes in personality and behavior gradually occur. The person will also complain of severe headaches and frequently exhibit epileptic convulsions.

To diagnose the cause of the problem, a general physical examination should be performed, including a neurological evaluation. Observation of the likely places where infection can start — the paranasal sinuses, mastoids, lungs, or heart (in individuals who have heart disease, which allows the shunting of infectious material through abnormal openings into the circulation of the brain) — aids in recognizing the sites of brain infection. Blood tests, both to make cultures and to see how the white blood cells are responding to the infection, are helpful. The most important test is usually a spinal puncture, which allows direct culture of the spinal fluid, and microscopic examination to see if any organisms can be recognized. Also, it's then possible to look at the cells in the spinal fluid and find whether or not spinal fluid chemistries are normal.

Therapies for Brain Infections

Once an infection has been diagnosed, specific therapies are undertaken in the most vigorous fashion. If the infection is bacterial, the appropriate antibiotic or combination of antibiotics must be administered promptly. If the infection is viral, antiviral medications can be given, although it should be pointed out that some viral agents don't respond well to medications, and moreover, some of the medications used to treat viral infections are themselves toxic and must be given with great care. Specific agents also exist to treat infections by spirochetes, as well as fungi.

I'd like to insert a word of caution here about the unrestricted use of spinal puncture before a complete neurological examination is done, including an ophthalmoscopic examination through the eyeball of the optic nerve head. If the optic disc is swollen, it may mean that there is increased pressure in the head, in which case a CAT scan or MRI examination of the brain should be performed before any spinal fluid is obtained by a spinal puncture. This routine serves as a precaution so that if a localized mass is present in the brain, such as a brain abscess, a protective cushion of spinal fluid will not be removed by a spinal puncture, allowing a portion of the brain mass to herniate against the brain stem.

Brain Abscesses

An abscess or localized brain infection is common enough that we should always keep the possibility in mind, even in persons who seem to exhibit the more generalized signs of brain infection. Most abscesses have to be evacuated and drained surgically or completely excised; only a few in the earliest stages can be successfully treated by massive antibiotic therapy.

Robert, twenty, a truck driver, was a muscular man who came to the hospital with a draining right ear and an infection of his middle ear and mastoid. He was immediately admitted when his neck became very stiff and he had an epileptic seizure. Following treatment, Robert recovered from the seizure, but he continued to have an intermittent spiking temperature and was confused and irrational at times. He also had a loss of recent memory. Over the course of several weeks, his vital memory deteriorated to the point that he recklessly broke social taboos by urinating in his bed and repeatedly masturbating in the open ward. He was belligerent as well, striking out at anyone who tried to examine or treat him.

Radio-opaque dye was injected into the major artery going to Robert's brain on the side of his draining ear, and x rays were taken as the dye traveled through the blood vessels of his brain. These x rays showed that Robert had a large abscess in the front end of his temporal lobe. Once the abscess was excised surgically his symptoms began to abate. The surgical excision was accompanied by effective treatment with antibiotics, which killed the offending bacterial organisms. Not only did Robert get back his vital memory, but his entire mental function soon returned to normal.

Physicians don't always do a spinal puncture in evaluating patients whose memory faculties and intellectual abilities are deteriorating, but perhaps they should, as the case of Jeremy, a sixty-three-year-old middle school teacher, illustrates. Jeremy had suffered a progressive loss of memory and was thought to be in the beginning stages of Alzheimer's disease. In the hospital, the results of all blood and urine tests, a medical examination, the CAT scan of his brain, and a brain wave test were within normal limits. He was discharged, yet his mental decline continued. Jeremy had to come to the hospital a second time before a lumbar puncture was carried out. The subsequent examination of his spinal fluid showed that it contained fungi and that he had a fungal infection around the base of his brain. The treatment of this infection brought some improvement, but he had residual memory loss that prevented him from being fully effective as a teacher, and he had to retire. His retirement would have been unnecessary if his problem had been diagnosed earlier.

Fungal infections of the brain and meninges are uncommon, but they can occur in anyone with an immune system deficiency, as in patients with AIDS. It is important to treat these infections early, and a spinal fluid exam should be done in every case of dementia that cannot be explained by routine testing.

Syphilitic Brain Infection

Two diseases that are sexually transmitted or spread through blood contact can produce late-onset infections of the brain, with resultant loss of memory and other intellectual functions. These only superficially similar diseases are syphilis and AIDS. Produced by a spirochete called treponema, syphilis progresses in three distinct phases: first, the primary chancre appears, usually on the genitals; a secondary outbreak of lesions can be in the mouth; finally, after five, ten, fifteen, even twenty years or more, an infection of the spinal cord, brain, or of the great vessels of the heart occurs. Although it is relatively uncommon today, syphilis of the brain used to fill the insane asylums and state mental hospitals with infected patients in the early part of this century.

Charlie, who was in the wholesale grocery business, was a patient of my father's who contracted syphilis about twenty years before I saw him. During my father's time, of course, there was no such thing as penicillin, and my father treated Charlie with drugs compounded from arsenic and with bismuth, and he gave him injections over a period of four or five years in the hope of eradicating the infection. My father was assiduous in checking for any problems in his patient's heart vessels, but Charlie didn't show signs of heart trouble, nor did he have another common complication of syphilis, tabes dorsalis, a syphilitic infection of the spinal cord. He did, however, develop syphilis of the brain.

I saw Charlie after my father died, when Charlie was sixty-seven years old. He had begun to have unusual changes in his moods, swinging from depression to unpredictable outbreaks of rage. He had always been a rather mild-mannered individual, and his sister, who lived with him, became deathly frightened when he started to threaten her. He also told me that he was having difficulty with his memory, and that his intellectual abilities had declined so that he was afraid he was making mistakes in his business.

Since my father's old records showed that many years before Charlie had had syphilis, I drew some blood to test for syphilis. But although the blood test was negative, Charlie's symptoms persisted. Just to be on the safe side, I decided to do a spinal puncture. I drew some spinal fluid and sent it to the state laboratory. Unlike the blood sample, the spinal fluid proved to be positive for syphilis, and I started treating Charlie with what was then a new drug, penicillin.

Oddly enough, a lot of doctors at first didn't have much confidence in penicillin for the treatment of syphilis, although of course over time it proved to be of immense value. Eventually Charlie's mental problems and his failing memory improved quite dramatically, and repeated examinations of his spinal fluid showed that he was free from syphilitic infection.

AIDS and Memory Loss

Autoimmune deficiency syndrome (AIDS) attacks the ability of the body's immune system to ward off disease, but it can also cause infections of the brain. At first we didn't realize that the brain, along with the immune system, is a primary target for the AIDS virus because the attack on the immune system produces all sorts of bizarre infections, some of which metastasize to the brain. It also makes patients susceptible to certain tumors or cancers, which invade the brain, and causes brain hemorrhages in some patients. Moreover, an individual infected with the AIDS virus can get a transient infection of the meninges, the tissues around the brain, after which the person may be asymptomatic for months or even years.

Researchers originally believed that all these brain problems were secondary to the assault on the immune system. However, AIDS patients often seemed unusually depressed and apathetic, and they had a noticeable reduction in intellectual ability and recent memory without showing focal lesions in the brain. We learned that these symptoms were due not to depression, but to an infestation of the brain by the AIDS virus itself which blocked the action of certain essential neurotransmitters.

Kevin was a skillful anesthesiologist at one of the hospitals where I worked. He became increasingly worried when some of his homosexual contacts developed clinical symptoms of AIDS. Then a blood test showed that he himself was positive for the AIDS virus. Initially Kevin became somewhat depressed and couldn't function very well. A CAT scan revealed brain atrophy, particularly in the front part of his brain.

Unhappily for Kevin, AZT had not yet been developed as a drug treatment for AIDS. His mental deterioration progressed rapidly, and subsequent CAT scans showed continuing alarming shrinkage of his brain. Kevin committed suicide less than a year before the drug AZT became available for treating AIDS. Only ten months after Kevin's suicide, in fact, we used AZT in treating a twenty-seven-year-old Haitian nurse who had an AIDS infection of the brain, dementia, and loss of recent memory, and she experienced a remarkable return of her intellectual abilities. Of course, AZT is not a cure for AIDS, and the improvement is temporary. Nevertheless, the improvement may last for several years with effective continued treatment.*

What to Look For in Brain Infections and How to Get Help

Brain infections can produce adverse changes in mental abilities, with major decreases in recent and other aspects of vital memory, through direct infestation of the brain, through consequent epileptic seizures, or through the delirium associated with infection. Overwhelming acute brain infections are easily diagnosed, but as I mentioned earlier, some persons

*Presently there are more powerful medications for the treatment of AIDS.

with smoldering brain infections may be misdiagnosed as having dementia or even depression. One physician prescribed electro-shock treatments for a very apathetic seamstress who was misdiagnosed as suffering from depression. When we did a spinal tap, our examination of her spinal fluid showed that she had bacterial meningitis, which was successfully treated with antibiotics.

The same rules for diagnosing other causes of memory loss — obtaining a good history and making thorough physical and laboratory examinations — also hold in diagnosing brain infection. Because some infections, if untreated, have a rapid and even fatal course, it is necessary to diagnose them with great dispatch.

With chronic infections, or those that progress slowly over weeks or months, we must exercise greater vigilance and suspicion, especially when these infections invade the inner portions of the temporal lobes, interfering with the memory process. The mood changes caused by some chronic infections mimic psychiatric problems and dementia. Patients are misdiagnosed as being severely depressed when, in fact, their problem is caused by direct brain infection. Diagnostic caution is especially called for in cases of tertiary syphilis as well as in some of the newer threats we all face, such as AIDS. Finally, we must not rule out brain infections such as syphilis as the cause of dementia and memory loss in elderly patients. Again, a spinal fluid examination may be critical in confirming the diagnosis.

The most important factor to consider with respect to brain infections is their prevention. Childhood immunization for measles also obviously prevents the complication of measles encephalitis. Prompt treatment of infections in other parts of the body, such as mastoid and sinus infections, will avert their spread to the brain. In areas of endemic encephalitis, avoiding mosquito bites by not going out at night, when mosquitoes are abundant, or using copious amounts of mosquito repellants is also wise. As far as diseases like AIDS and syphilis are concerned, avoiding sexual promiscuity and, in the former case, avoiding the sharing of needles among intravenous drug users are critical in preventing brain infection.

As fast as we develop new antibiotics and methods of immunization, ever more exotic infectious agents seem to appear on the medical scene. Some of these can be found in hospital settings, and even in blood banks. Every area of medical practice — hospitals, clinics, blood banks — must therefore continue to use the most scrupulous care to avoid transmitting infectious agents, particularly those that can cause damage to our vital memory functions.

Vital Memory Points to Remember

1. Brain infections can be caused by bacteria, fungi, protozoans, and viruses, all of which can produce memory loss.
2. A brain abscess is a localized brain infection that can result in confusion, irritability, memory loss, seizures, and signs of increased pressure in the brain.
3. Sexually transmitted diseases and diseases carried by blood, including AIDS, produce a variety of brain infections, all of which can cause memory loss.

16

Closed-Head Injuries and Memory Loss

IN MY MEDICAL PRACTICE I've seen literally hundreds of patients with closed-head injuries that resulted in mild to severe loss of memory. The vast majority of these injuries were caused by automobile collisions. Because some people walk away from car crashes without realizing how badly they've been injured, it sometimes takes weeks before the resulting loss of brain function is reported. Quite often it is not even the victim but rather a close friend or relative who recognizes the loss of memory function and encourages the patient to seek medical treatment. Indeed, closed-head injuries may produce such a prolonged decline in memory and mental abilities that even the reluctant patient will finally agree that medical treatment is the only viable course of action.

Because the brain is a semigelatinous mass with a cushion of spinal fluid around and within it, suspended on a fountain of blood within the bony box that is the cranium, it can withstand most minor bumps and bruises without ill effect. But any acceleration or deceleration accident whose impact exceeds the elasticity of the brain and the cushioning effect of the spinal fluid will damage the base of the frontal lobes and the tips of the temporal lobes. In addition, if there is twisting or turning of the head, tearing of the axons, the nerve fibers leading impulses away from the brain cells, may occur.

The injuries I've just described are different from open-head injuries, in which there is a penetrating wound of the brain. Being hit by a bullet or a baseball bat, for example, causes a depressed fracture of the skull, with bone slivers penetrating the membranes of the brain and actually sticking into the brain itself. Open-head injuries obviously cause brain damage, and often secondary epileptic seizures, because of their direct effect on brain tissue. But the closed-head injury, in which no penetration of the skull occurs, can also wreak destructive effects in the front part of the brain and on the internal fibers of the brain.

The complications of both closed- and open-head injuries are magnified in the elderly. The brains of older persons have fewer brain cells and lesser redundancy, so that any loss of function is less apt to be compensated for by recircuiting through another, uninjured pathway, such as occurs in a younger individual or especially in a child. Also, the smaller volume of the brains of elderly persons makes their brains more susceptible to tears of blood vessels in angular, decelerating brain injuries.

The Three Kinds of Closed-Head Injuries

Closed-head injuries fall into three categories: major, minor, and trivial. Major head injuries, which require hospitalization for more than twenty-four hours, result in loss of consciousness or memory for more than twenty to forty minutes and of course produce prolonged loss of brain function. Minor head injuries, treated during a hospital stay of less than twenty-four hours, produce a loss of consciousness or memory for less than twenty minutes. But the fact that a head injury is deemed minor does not make it insignificant. Trivial head injuries are the kind children often get when they bump their heads. No real injury to the brain itself occurs because the cushioning effect of the spinal fluid and the absorption of the energy of impact by the scalp and skull prevent damage to underlying brain tissue.

Most head injuries (except in the elderly, who are more at risk than the young) are of the trivial variety and need not concern us. We are concerned here with the so-called minor head injuries that turn out to be not so minor. They are not only associated with memory problems lasting anywhere from four to six weeks, but also with difficulties in social adjustment, marital harmony, and work performance as well as with depression that may endure for many months and even years. When these complications of minor head injuries are superimposed on a heart or liver condition, for example, which many people in their seventies or eighties may have, their effects prove to be minor only in comparison with those of the life-threatening and devastating major head injuries. In addition, even mild head injuries in the elderly can have late complications such as subdural hematomas.

Carlos was a sixty-year-old jazz musician who played various kinds of electric guitars. One night the members of his band finished work late, after public transportation had stopped running, and so Carlos asked one of the band members to drive him home. When he was dropped off he tried to leave the car quickly, but in doing so he accidentally closed the car door on his coat. When the car suddenly accelerated, Carlos was upended and bounced along the highway, on his head, for about twenty-five feet before his anguished cry caused the driver of the car to stop.

Although he was dazed and briefly lost his memory of some of the events that occurred at the time of his injury, examinations at the hospital did not disclose any skull fracture, and Carlos was sent home. Headaches, difficulty with recent memory, inability to plan, a lack of initiative, and a complete disintegration of his work-related activities persisted for some months after his head injury.

When it became obvious that he could no longer perform at his previous level, Carlos sought medical help. A complete neurological evaluation showed some abnormalities in the neuropsychological exam and in the computerized brain wave test. But these were minor compared with the social and functional impairment Carlos suffered. This man was not having seizures and was not an alcohol or drug abuser. I noted that he was clearly depressed, which is common after a minor brain injury. And, of course, depression may have exacerbated his problems with recent memory.

Treatment of the depression, along with large doses of tincture of time, was the prescription that worked in Carlos's case. It took almost two years before he returned to the same level of activity he had engaged in before his head injury, but he did recover fully.

Disability After a Minor Head Injury

The clinical course of chronic disability after a minor head or brain injury is all too common. The patient has objective signs of memory loss which clear up after four to six weeks, but is then left with disabling depression, headache, changes in mood and behavior, difficulty in social interactions, trouble in performing any kind of job, and increasing friction and tension in domestic relationships. From my own experience and reports in the literature on head injuries, I would judge that there may be more than a hundred thousand patients a year who suffer minor head or brain injuries, chiefly in automobile accidents, and whose course is similar to that of Carlos. All too often cases of this sort end up in court, usually because the representatives of insurance companies don't believe that minor head injuries can be so disabling. A small percentage of these patients injure their heads at work, in which case they come up in review before workers' compensation boards. The issue of financial compensation by insurance companies in cases of prolonged disability has been subjected to intense scrutiny. But although the precise cause of disability is often not agreed on, there is no question that such disability stemming from head injuries is genuine. It is not a "compensation neurosis" — that is, a problem with physical symptoms which disappear once a settlement is reached.

Amnesia and Closed-Head Injuries

The immediate consequences of head injury may be retrograde amnesia, in which the victim has difficulty recalling events that preceded the brain injury, or antrograde amnesia, in which the victim blocks out for a matter of minutes to hours, or sometimes even days, the events following a head injury.

That's what happened to Karen, a fifty-seven-year-old instructor, who was sitting in the passenger seat of an automobile struck head-on by a drunken driver speeding in the wrong lane. She was unconscious for a time following the injury and was in the hospital for several weeks. She then began to make a gradual recovery, to the extent that six months later she returned to teaching. Karen then found that her ability to study and teach was compromised, which clearly signaled memory problems since the recent-memory function is central to the acquisition of new information — that is, to learning. Karen had to transfer many of her students to other teachers and dropped down to limited teaching.

She sued the drunken driver, but when the case went to trial, the insurance company covering the other driver minimized Karen's problems, saying that because she was able to teach in a college, she couldn't have suffered major brain injury. It was at this point that we undertook a full evaluation of Karen's case, including neuropsychological and psychodiagnostic tests as well as brain wave studies, neurological examinations, and a CAT scan of the brain. Karen's brain examinations showed a previously unsuspected hole inside her brain which had been caused by the destruction of brain tissue at the time of the accident. This loss of brain tissue resulted in her loss of memory.

Karen's case has two important lessons. First, even patients over fifty who have had major brain injuries may recover a significant amount of their mental abilities, so that inexperienced observers may say that they are completely normal when they are not. And second, even when such recovery takes place, a full neurological evaluation is necessary to pinpoint residual problems. This is important not only in working out programs for future rehabilitation but also in determining the amount of functional loss. When Karen's loss was presented to a jury, she was compensated with over $3 million in damages.

In my experience, neither the patient nor the physician should ever give up hope of recovery after a serious head injury. The mental abilities of one of my patients, a sixty-three-year-old man who had experienced severe intellectual deterioration and memory loss after a major head injury, were significantly restored *five years* after the damage to his brain occurred. Such improvement is more likely in a closed- than in an open-head injury because extreme loss of brain tissue is less common in patients who suffer closed-head injury.

Seat Belts, Air Bags, and Head Injuries

Every year, as many as half a million persons in the United States injure their brains as a result of automobile collisions. Of the fifty thousand or more people who die in automobile accidents, seventy percent of the deaths are due directly to brain injury. Some other victims who survive are so severely brain-injured and have lost so much of their vital memories that they will spend the rest of their lives in chronic care institutions. Many of the others with less serious injuries will substantially recover. Even so, they may have lost some brain function if their injuries have caused a loss of brain tissue, which cannot regenerate.

The clear message from all these facts is the importance of prevention. If every automobile in the United States were equipped with three-point shoulder and lap restraints, plus air bags for every passenger, most of these brain injuries and deaths would be averted.* This solution is expensive, of course — but it is even more expensive to care for chronically disabled brain-injured patients who will remain in nursing homes for the rest of their lives. Finally, we must consider more than just the expenditure of money. We also have to think of the waste of human potential and the interruption of useful lives which are a consequence of brain injury. This effect is magnified in the elderly, who tolerate brain injury to a lesser extent than do younger persons.

It is within our power to exert the political and moral persuasion that will reduce or prevent most brain injuries, through an educational campaign directed at the president of the United States and the U.S. Congress. Congress should legislate national safety standards for every car and truck on the road, which would virtually eliminate the occurrence of the majority of serious brain injuries. That such legislation has not yet been passed is a national tragedy.

Vital Memory Points to Remember
1. Closed-head injuries are most often caused by automobile accidents.
2. Even so-called minor head injuries can result in difficulties with mental functioning and memory for months and years.
3. Half a million persons injure their heads as a result of car collisions in the United States each year. One hundred thousand of these injuries are serious.
4. Installation of air bags in cars and use of three-point shoulder restraints would greatly reduce the severity of head injuries sustained in accidents.

*Air bags are now redesigned to avoid injury to children.

17

Epilepsy and Memory Loss

HAVE YOU EVER SEEN someone have an epileptic seizure? Do you think that people who have epilepsy are different from you and me? If you do, you're wrong; anyone, you and me included, could have a seizure if our brains were subjected to sufficient injury or toxic exposure. Contrary to what you may have thought, epilepsy is actually a symptom rather than a disease, characterized by episodic alterations in consciousness related to electrical abnormalities in the brain. Anyone, I would like to reiterate, if given enough brain poisons like alcohol or cocaine, can have an epileptic seizure, although individuals with a family predisposition to seizures may have a lower threshold for them than the average person. And, of course, seizures can be provoked not only by brain poisons but also by brain tumors, brain injuries, strokes, and brain infections.

What many people often forget is that epileptic seizures can be either generalized or localized. There are two kinds of generalized seizures. The grand mal seizure, the classic major seizure, is associated with complete loss of consciousness, breath holding, urinary incontinence, tongue biting, fixed posture and alternating contraction of the muscles, and stertorous breathing (a heavy snoring sound), whereas the petit mal seizure, which is most often seen in children, brings about just small lapses in consciousness.

A localized, or partial, epileptic seizure can start at any area of the brain which is irritated, producing a seizure related to a specific brain structure. A seizure in the motor area, for instance, can cause an epileptic movement in a hand or the side of the mouth; in the sensory area of the brain, it can produce sensations. These partial seizures can become generalized, or they can remain local.

If seizures occur in the emotional or limbic part of the brain, the area associated with the laying down of new memories, they are known as partial complex seizures. These spells can start with the hallucination of a bad smell or bad taste, or a funny feeling in the abdomen. They are succeeded by chewing movements and occasionally automatic behavior — that is, making an inappropriate movement again and again. Partial complex seizures may also develop into generalized seizures. Sometimes just a fragment of the seizure is observable — the "aura" or warning, such as a bad taste or smell, or a blank stare on the face of the patient for just a few moments.

Some of my patients who experienced this kind of seizure became belligerent during and immediately before or after the seizure. But most often belligerence, excessive religiosity, forced writing, and a profound lack of sexual drive were seen between seizures rather than during the episodes themselves. Such changes are rare in epilepsy originating in the nonemotional parts of the brain.

Partial Complex Seizures and Memory Loss

Because limbic or partial complex seizures so often begin in the anterior medial part of the temporal lobes, in close proximity to important parts of the memory circuit, loss of memory is a frequent consequence, one that often manifests itself clinically in periods of confusion. And if an individual has repeated small seizures, loss of memory may be so intense that long-lasting confusion results.

Very occasionally, seizures produce loss of memory for a length of time during which the patient engages in rather complicated but appropriate behavior. Such was the case with Fred, twenty-eight, an ex-marine who had a small shrapnel wound in one of his temporal lobes, the scar of which generated partial complex seizures.

After Fred got out of the Marine Corps on disability, he took a job driving a tractor-trailer between Reno and Los Angeles. He described episodes of having these little blackout spells just outside Reno and coming to his senses as he was nearing the truck depot in Los Angeles. Incredibly, Fred would have no idea of how he got from one place to the other, although on one occasion a relief driver who was with him swore that he did everything perfectly, drove safely, and completed his run on time.

When Fred consulted me about his seizures, he was obviously quite disturbed. Even though we were able to reduce the number of his seizures and the resultant memory loss by the use of antiseizure medication, he quit truck driving and became an electrician: "It was just too nerve-racking," he explained.

Epileptic Seizures in Older Individuals

At times an epileptic seizure may be the first symptom of a problem of the brain needing urgent attention. Generalized seizures are easy to recognize, but partial seizures can too readily be missed, particularly when they occur in an older individual. They may be misdiagnosed as Alzheimer's disease or some other incurable and progressive ailment, or as simply a loss of function with old age. Misdiagnosis is especially regrettable when memory loss, periods of confusion, and seeming dementia are caused by seizures, since they are readily treatable and the memory loss they cause can be reversed.

Epileptic Seizures and Alzheimer's

If seizures occur at all in Alzheimer's disease, they happen very late in the progress of the disorder, when intellectual loss is advanced and recent and remote memory are nil. Seizures usually do not occur early in the course of the disease, and therefore when patients have seizures and their main problem is loss of memory, without any great loss of intellectual capacity, it is quite unlikely that the correct diagnosis is Alzheimer's disease.

Because they abnormally block memory pathways, seizures can produce confusional states and loss of memory without any other brain disease being present. Small, repeated seizures that are difficult to discern can cause long-lasting loss of memory, which is hard to differentiate from memory loss resulting from other causes, such as tiny strokes or the beginning stages of Alzheimer's disease.

Detecting Epileptic Seizures

Finally, you should be aware that some seizures cannot be detected, even by brain wave tests, especially when the seizures occur deep within the brain — such as, for example, near certain sensitive parts of the memory circuits. Partial complex seizures, or minor seizures, may occur in the depths of the brain while surface recordings show normal brain wave activity. This fact makes it all the more difficult to establish a positive and accurate diagnosis, and repeated examinations, including twenty-four-hour brain wave recordings, are often necessary. Even so, these sophisticated examinations may still miss small seizures that disrupt memory function and produce confusion, and patients suspected of having such seizures are therefore sometimes given a therapeutic trial of antiseizure medication.

Any past history of brain trauma, brain infection, or childhood or febrile convulsions, or a family history of seizures, should increase your awareness of this possible cause of periods of confusion and memory loss. You should know too that strokes and brain hemorrhages may also produce electrical disturbances and seizures. And, of course, any kind of structural brain abnormality seen on a CAT or MRI scan, such as a brain tumor or arteriovenous malformation, can also generate a seizure disorder. Keep in mind, however, that although structural abnormalities can increase the tendency to have seizures, no matter whether an epileptic seizure or convulsion is generalized or partial, it is a functional disturbance of the brain. Temporary or prolonged memory loss and confusion are frequently the result.

Great advances have been made in the treatment of epilepsy by medication. Tracey Putnam, a neurosurgeon who preceded me at the Boston City Hospital, discovered the effectiveness of Dilantin in preventing seizures in the 1930s. This agent was the first to stop seizures without producing sedation. Partial complex seizures have similarly been helped by the use of another medicine called Tegretol, and attacks of petit mal epilepsy have been reduced in frequency by valproic acid medications. Occasionally, when these or other medications don't work, the surgical removal of an epileptic focus will eliminate seizures. Through reduction or elimination of seizures, the confusion and memory loss that accompany them can also be reversed.

Vital Memory Points to Remember

1. Epilepsy is a symptom, not a disease.
2. If given enough brain poisons, anyone can have an epileptic seizure.
3. Memory loss is common during epileptic seizures.
4. Once diagnosed, memory loss caused by seizures can be restored once the seizures are stopped.

18

Strokes and Memory Loss

You MAY HAVE the notion that all patients with strokes are paralyzed and that there's not much you can do for them, but that notion is wrong. The symptoms of some stroke patients can be reversed with treatment. Rehabilitation therapies can improve the condition of many stroke victims and, of course, many strokes can be prevented by reducing fats in the diet and by effectively treating high blood pressure.

There are various kinds of stroke, many of which can bring about memory loss. Not all strokes are the same, and what's more, their treatments are not the same. Major strokes are of two varieties: those related to rupturing of a blood vessel, leading to brain hemorrhage; and those related to the closing off or plugging up of a blood vessel by an embolus or arteriosclerotic occlusion. This shuts off the flow of blood through the vessel, depriving an area of the brain of its blood supply and killing the affected segment of brain tissue. This is called a cerebral infarct.

Major infarcts are announced at times by blindness or paralysis that lasts for a few minutes and then goes away. These temporary strokes, called transient ischemic attacks, are caused by tiny platelet emboli from ulcers in the carotid artery in the neck — or by incomplete closure of the brain's blood vessels. They are often a warning that a major stroke is on the way, and prompt treatment is necessary, such as surgery to remove arteriosclerotic plaques from the diseased carotid artery. The operation, called a carotid endarterectomy, is often effective in preventing further trouble. Even when the source of a stroke is a hemorrhage instead of an infarct, surgical removal of the hemorrhage is often possible, depending on its location and cause.

Multi-Infarct Dementia

Surprisingly, because they are often multiple, small or tiny strokes are a frequent cause of memory loss and intellectual and mood changes, producing a syndrome called multi-infarct dementia. In one variety of this disorder, patients' small blood vessels in their brains are fairly normal but the large blood vessels in their necks, such as the carotids, have blood vessel disease, or the patients may have abnormal areas in the linings of their hearts. These areas are predisposed to clot formation and small clots or parts of clots may break off, forming emboli that travel to the smaller tiny blood vessels of the brain, where they block the vessels and produce small infarcts, or strokes. As can be seen in the case of Hattie, the clinical pattern of these strokes is characteristic.

Hattie was the sixty-seven-year-old matriarch of a large family, and three of her daughters as well as many grandchildren lived with her. She was a God-fearing, hard-working woman who held a full-time job in a factory, kept the family accounts, and was extremely responsible.

One morning Hattie's oldest daughter found her wandering around her bedroom, seemingly dazed and confused. When the daughter told her that she would be late for work, she couldn't seem to focus on the words, and she made no attempt to get dressed. Hattie's daughter called her employer and told him that her mother was sick and couldn't come in — which in itself was unusual since Hattie hadn't missed a day of work

215

in decades. For the next three or four days, although her confusion persisted, she seemed to recover little by little. When a week had passed she seemed ready to get on with her life.

But Hattie's mental powers weren't quite as good as they had been before. She wasn't as alert or as focused. She knew generally what she had to do, but she wasn't the sharp executive who ran the entire family so efficiently. Gradually her daughters took over a fair amount of responsibility. Life went on for another six or seven weeks, and then the same thing happened all over again, except that this time her confusional period and memory loss lasted a little longer and her recovery was even less perfect.

I hear this kind of story often from people with multi-infarct dementia. They have small strokes, often occurring deep inside the brain and in a variable pattern, which reduce recent memory and seem to be progressive. Some victims of this disease are misdiagnosed as having Alzheimer's. And, of course, when they go to their doctors, they're told that there's nothing that can be done for them, and no further investigation of possible causes of their problem is made.

Some researchers think that multi-infarct dementia is always caused by the closing off of very tiny blood vessels in the brain — that is, small arteries. But an astute neuropathologist who did post-mortem examinations on multi-infarct dementia patients who died failed to find much evidence of primary blood vessel disease. He has postulated that sometimes the disease is caused by little clots that break off from the great vessels in the neck which go to the brain, or from the lining of the heart itself, or from a diseased valve of the heart. This theory, if confirmed, has practical significance because medicines (including aspirin) that thin the blood and reduce clotting may prevent the recurrence of this problem. Depending on the site at which the clots originate, surgical treatment may also be helpful.

Tests for Diagnosing
Multi-Infarct Dementia (Type I)

Anthony, a fifty-seven-year-old ranch worker, had been complaining of feeling faint and having difficulty with recent memory. He went to see a neurosurgeon because an article in the local newspaper had told about some remarkable surgical treatment that helped people with just his symptoms. The article stated that local hardening of the arteries in the great vessels of the neck narrowed the blood vessels to such an extent that a noise resulted as the blood rushed by the area of partial obstruction. It furthermore stated that to screen for this problem, a doctor could put a stethoscope to the patient's neck and would be able to hear the noise of the blood passing through the constricted area.

Besides feeling faint and showing signs of memory failure, Anthony had been hearing a funny noise in one ear. So he looked up the neurosurgeon mentioned in the newspaper article and made an urgent appointment. When the doctor listened at his neck he heard a striking bruit corresponding to the noise Anthony himself heard.

All this took place before the invention of CAT scans and magnetic resonance imaging. The neurosurgeon made extensive x-ray tests, placing a small catheter in the great vessels carrying arterial blood to the brain and injecting these vessels with radio-opaque solutions that could be visualized by x rays as the solution went through the blood vessels. In this way he followed the course of the radio-opaque solution from the base of the neck all the way up to the brain.

Fortunately for Anthony, his partial blockage occurred in only one of his carotid arteries at the point where it branched into the internal and external divisions. Surgical treatment required opening the artery and carefully removing the arteriosclerotic plaque that obstructed the passage, making certain

217

that no little clots broke off and deposited themselves in the brain.

Anthony seemed to be perfectly all right, with good neurological function, in the immediate postoperative period. But about six hours later he began to feel weakness in one arm and his lower face, on the side opposite to where the operation had been performed. The surgeon thought the clot might have recurred at the site of the operation and that he might have to go in and remove it. But first he elevated Anthony's blood pressure, and the partial paralysis disappeared. The doctor had to keep the blood pressure elevated for about three days, then gradually allowed it to drift back to normal. Anthony had no further symptoms, and he was able to go back to work without any problems. More important, he did not have any episodes of tiny strokes caused by the breaking off of little clots or groups of platelets from the diseased artery because the anatomical site that could harbor clots and potential emboli had been completely removed.

Ultrasound of the heart and of the great blood vessels in the neck may be helpful in determining which of the possible sites of embolic strokes is at fault. In addition, x rays following the injection of radio-opaque substances into the blood stream as well as specialized MRI scans may help locate the site of the problem in the blood vessels and heart. And of course today CAT scans and magnetic resonance images of the brain can establish the clinical diagnosis of multi-infarct dementia anatomically.

An important message I want to convey is not to take the diagnosis of Alzheimer's disease as final until a very thorough and accurate history has been taken. If a person with decreasing memory has had episodes of confusion, with gradual improvement until the next episode, the problem is probably not Alzheimer's disease but multi-infarct dementia produced by these tiny repeated strokes. The great tragedy is that if this condition is left untreated and future strokes are not prevented, so many tiny strokes will occur that deep and irreversible dementia will result. These may be severe enough to irreparably impair vital memory. It is possible, however, to treat such patients and prevent future problems if the disease is found early enough. The following case is an illustration.

Alfred was the owner of a small dry-cleaning business, who had a long history of heart disease with auricular fibrillation. When I saw him in one of the local Boston hospitals, he had an uneven gait and some loss of memory. In addition, other mental abilities were interfered with to the point that he could not run his business. A CAT scan taken in the course of his neurological evaluation showed tiny little strokes in the deep and superficial parts of his brain. This scan was made with one of the first CAT scanners to be set up in the northeastern United States, and the pictures were not as clear as those made by today's CAT scanners. But the diagnosis was unmistakable, and Alfred was put on blood thinners at age fifty-five.

I followed Alfred's case for twelve years. He recovered some of his mental powers, had no progression of his disease, and was able to function quite adequately with his wife in the dry-cleaning business until they sold it and retired to Florida.

The lesson is that the clinical picture of anyone with memory loss and other kinds of mental deterioration, along with loss of sensation or vision, weakness of an arm or a leg, or impaired coordination on one side, points to multi-infarct dementia rather than Alzheimer's disease, and the progression of this disorder can be arrested by anticoagulant treatment.

Finally, multi-infarct dementia, just like Alzheimer's, can be made much worse by depression, malnutrition, or brain poisoning with various sedative or psychiatric drugs as well as alcohol and street drugs like cocaine. Cocaine itself can produce tiny or large strokes even in young people who have no history of arterial disease or prior heart problems.

Multi-Infarct Dementia (Type II): Border Zone Infarct

In what is known as Binswanger's disease, or border zone infarct, another kind of tiny stroke occurs in the border zones of the brain when there isn't enough blood pressure to force the arterial blood through partially obstructed arteries. Persons taking an excess amount of antihypertensive medication can be susceptible to these strokes, particularly when they stand up and become hypotensive — that is, their blood pressure drops below normal levels.

If the periods of low blood pressure are long enough, tiny strokes occur in the inside part of the brain. The areas in which these strokes occur are the so-called watershed or border zones, which derive their name from the fact that they are located in the deep areas of the brain at the border between the part of the brain supplied by one artery (for example, the anterior cerebral artery) and a part of the brain supplied by another (the middle cerebral artery). The border zones are only marginally supplied by both arteries, and when a decrease in blood pressure results in decreased irrigation of blood through the brain, they may not get enough blood, producing a small stroke, or infarct. Disease of the small vessels of the brain, the penetrating blood vessels, is also often present.

Many doctors do not distinguish between the tiny strokes that occur in the border zones of the brain in Binswanger's disease and those that produce multi-infarct dementia type I, although I believe the two are quite separate entities. Taken together, these two stroke-producing conditions are frequent causes of lost intellectual function and memory loss. This is not only true in nursing home patients but also in people living independently at home. It's therefore essential that anyone whose intellectual or memory abilities have declined seek competent medical attention promptly and have a thorough evaluation to rule out these disorders, since these are problems that can be treated and prevented.

Blood Pressure: High and Low

One factor that has led to a great reduction in the incidence of strokes has been doctors' recognition that people with uncontrolled high blood pressure are much more likely to suffer strokes than people with normal blood pressure. Because of the beneficial effects of keeping blood pressure within normal limits, many doctors prescribe antihypertensive agents if patients have one or two blood pressure readings above accepted normal limits. They seem to think it is better to err on the side of keeping the blood pressure low than to take a chance on future stroke.

But high blood pressure is not the only factor that contributes to strokes. The same dietary problems that are related to premature heart attacks, namely, diets too high in saturated fats, may also be related to disease of the blood vessels in the brain and subsequent strokes. Even if a stroke does not occur, the narrowing of a blood vessel may make it more susceptible to low blood pressure. There just isn't enough pressure in the arterial blood vessels to force the blood through the narrowed, diseased arteries for a normal irrigation of brain tissue. This problem is more common with the widespread use of antihypertensive agents, even in people under age fifty.

Greg was a forty-three-year-old accountant whose high-stress existence, especially around tax time, kept him in a state of continual anxiety. Because his blood pressure was high, his doctor put him on antihypertensive medication. The problem with Greg was that he thought that if one antihypertensive pill was good for him, two were twice as good — so when he felt under stress, he doubled up on his medication.

Because Greg didn't recognize what was happening to him, he inadvertently forced his blood pressure down below nor-

mal limits. He didn't pay attention to the warning signs —
particularly when he got up out of bed and felt dizzy and
unsteady, as if he was going to topple over.

Greg took enough medication during tax time that he
started to have lower-than-normal blood pressure even when
he wasn't standing up, and he began to notice that he was
unsteady when he walked. Worst of all, he began having difficulty with recent memory, and he appeared slowed down, depressed, and apathetic.

As an accomplished professional, Greg had always prided
himself on his good memory, and a good memory was necessary to assist the diverse clients who used his services, each
with their own individual and sometimes complicated problems. When he consulted me he was afraid he was getting
Alzheimer's disease. But what I saw when I took a CAT scan
of his brain tissue revealed quite a different picture. Because of
his self-induced low blood pressure, he had had tiny little
strokes in the border zones around the outer surface of the
fluid-filled spaces of his brain.

I put Greg on an antidepressant medicine called Desyrel and
referred him back to his internist for better control of his antihypertensive medication. Both his walking and his memory
improved dramatically, even though the small strokes seen on
his CAT scan stayed the same. The reason an antidepressant
like Desyrel works in cases like Greg's is that border zone
strokes destroy brain fibers that carry neurotransmitters. The
antidepressant stimulant helps make up for the neurotransmitter deficiency.

Binswanger's disease, microvascular infarctions in the border zones of the brain leading to loss of intellectual capacity, is
usually seen in people much older than Greg. Because CAT
scans of older patients sometimes show a decrease in the density of border zone tissues not accompanied by specific mental
changes, some doctors think the diagnosis of Binswanger's
disease is overused. I disagree. In fact my partner, Tom Sabin,

and his associate Gopal Venna have evidence that this syndrome, which is often made worse by antihypertensive drugs, is much more common than is generally recognized.

Controlling Your Own Blood Pressure

My point is to alert you to the fact that blood pressure should be neither too high nor too low. In no way do I mean to keep you from taking necessary medication to reduce high blood pressure, but it should be reserved for those who really need it. Some persons with mildly elevated blood pressure can be managed by diet alone — a diet not only low in fat but especially in saturated fat, and which also severely restricts salt (primarily sodium) intake.

Many of the foods you buy in the supermarket list the amount of sodium they contain on the labels. Read these labels. Going on a low-sodium diet requires more than just not putting added salt from a salt shaker on your food; it means avoiding many kinds of canned foods and soups that are simply loaded with sodium.

It's difficult to understand food producers who present items for sale which contain low amounts of salt but high amounts of saturated fats in the form of hydrogenated oil. Why would anyone who has to restrict intake of sodium want to buy low-salt peanut butter made with hydrogenated peanut oil? It doesn't make any sense nutritionally, and the manufacturers of such products should be educated to serve the best interests of the public by reducing not only sodium but also saturated and total fats in their products.

Another thing to remember about blood pressure level is that it may vary considerably depending on the level of exertion as well as the emotional state of the person being monitored. Some people get so anxious about the possibility of having high blood pressure that they actually send their blood pressure up when they are having it taken by a nurse or physician. It's important, obviously, to obtain a base-line reading for each patient. The art of getting a true reading, not a stressed one, may require considerable patience on the part of the medical care-giver.

Gwen, an amateur musician, had had rheumatic heart disease when she was sixteen, which produced a loud murmur. She always dreaded going to the doctor because she was afraid her heart was defective, and that the defect would be obvious to any physician who listened to her chest. Her usual doctor retired when she was fifty-two, and the new doctor who saw her was rather stiff and formal. Gwen became frightened when he took her blood pressure. It was 160. He had her come in again a week later, when it was even higher. It finally stabilized at 180; that's when he put her on antihypertensive medication, and one of the pills he gave her was the beta blocker propranolol. He also had her restrict her salt intake.

Gwen took the medication for six or seven months. During that time she felt more and more depressed and confused, and she was worried about her failing memory. Exasperated about her ill health, and without even asking her doctor, she stopped taking the medication but continued to restrict her salt intake. In a short time she felt much better and was much more alert, and her memory returned to normal.

Thirty years later, after she had moved to another state, Gwen broke her hip. She had her blood pressure taken a number of times, both before and after her hip replacement surgery and of course during the surgical procedure. Her blood pressure was absolutely normal, and it continued in the normal range until she died at the age of eighty-six.

The example of Gwen shows that if mild high blood pressure is treated in time (and if there is no kidney disease or diabetes), a low-salt diet may be adequate to prevent strokes. And, of course, blood pressure is unlikely to be too low when it is managed by diet alone.

Major Strokes and Memory Loss

In the popular mind, someone who has suffered a stroke becomes paralyzed on one side of the body, often with partial or total loss of speech. Indeed, many strokes present in just this way, but some instead result in a loss of a visual field, or of sensation in one part or one half of the body, as well as of intellectual and memory functions. Also, major strokes are sometimes correlated with major heart attacks, and it is not unusual for these two clinical problems to occur within six months of one another.

The factors that predispose a person to major stroke and heart attack are very similar. A genetic factor influences the way the body handles saturated fats and cholesterol, high blood pressure, and a high salt (sodium chloride) intake. Also, a diet rich in saturated fats, including such foods as pork, bacon, ham, tenderloin steaks, and often the tastiest cuts of meat (the taste is often in the saturated fat) as well as excessive amounts of butter, cream, ice cream, and whole milk (as opposed to skim milk), contributes to one's propensity for having either stroke or heart attack.

The list of foods high in saturated fats extends to hot dogs and hamburgers, some kinds of cheese, egg yolks, and many rich desserts such as cakes and pies made with vegetable shortening, lard, or hydrogenated oil. Combine this kind of diet with insufficient exercise, add some canned foods with high salt content, which increases the tendency toward high blood pressure, and just for good measure keep on smoking cigarettes, and you have a prescription for early heart attack and stroke, especially if your genetic makeup makes you predisposed to have such problems.

Memory loss can be the direct result of a stroke that involves the memory pathways, and particularly the inner parts of the temporal lobe. Millie, a seventy-six-year-old homemaker, had a single large stroke in one temporal lobe at age sixty-eight, and then some years later a second stroke in the opposite temporal lobe after surgery to remove one of her breasts. Her second stroke left her with the physical symptom of only mild weakness, but it devastated her mentally: she suffered a completely incapacitating loss of recent memory. In effect, her vital memory was irreversibly destroyed, and she existed in a kind of time warp, unable to remember any of her ongoing experiences. Her children were disturbed by her symptoms and thought she had become insane. It was not of much comfort to Millie, but we were able to show her bewildered relatives the CAT scans of her two strokes. They understood the origin of her disabling symptoms and were able to provide her with sympathetic and appropriate supportive treatment.

Things to Be Aware Of

Memory loss occurs in people who have had strokes for several independent reasons. The first is the death of brain tissue (infarction) containing portions of the memory pathways. Secondary effects of the stroke such as depression, brain intoxication with prescription drugs, or malnutrition stemming from incapacity may also cause memory loss.

Finally, a possible cause of memory loss related to stroke is epileptic seizure. Such a seizure may occur early, at the time of the initial insult to the brain, or later, as the infarct scars over and begins to irritate surrounding brain tissue, resulting in a convulsion. In some patients these epileptic seizures are obvious, whereas in others very localized seizures can be easily missed, even by a trained observer. The seizures can affect the functioning of the memory pathways, producing transient amnesia, and if they are repeated the amnesia can be quite prolonged. The problem is treatable by antiseizure medication.

The best treatment for stroke is prevention through watching the diet, exercising, maintaining normal blood pressure, and avoiding tobacco, alcohol, and other drugs like cocaine which can produce strokes. When a stroke has occurred, however, it is important to examine the stroke victim carefully to see if memory has been affected. Preservation of memory, and especially vital memory, can be an essential stepping stone for rehabilitating movement, speech, and even certain aspects of intelligence.

In the rehabilitation process it is also necessary to keep the attention of stroke patients focused on something or someone besides themselves. Directing attention to an outside problem is the best way to avert depression. Secondary depression in someone who has suffered a stroke can be almost as disabling, as far as impairing memory is concerned, as the stroke itself, and its reversal can help preserve vital memory.

A patient who has had a stroke should have a CAT or MRI scan done, which will define the precise part of brain tissue which has been lost and assess the structure of the remaining brain tissue in the area of the stroke. Such an assessment can give a picture of the parts of the brain which are still structurally sound and capable of taking over lost brain function with the aid of directed rehabilitation therapy.

Finally, even after restricting saturated fats and salt in your diet — and giving up smoking — you may require antihypertensive medicine prescribed by your physician. You should know, however, that not all of these medicines are equally safe or effective. Some antihypertensive drugs, called alpha blockers, not only lower blood pressure but also reduce the "bad" kinds of cholesterol in your blood. Get as much information as you can about the medicine you'll be taking before you start your treatment, and be aware of both the potential benefits and the side effects.

Since we published the first edition of this book in 1992, a number of medical studies have revealed new information about the incidence and prevention of strokes. Some of the studies, which are discussed below, may seem contradictory in their implications. However, it is important for you to see the new evidence, evaluate it, and then take action in a prudent fashion to safeguard your health.

One of the least controversial studies was produced by the department of ambulatory care and prevention at Harvard medical school in 1995. This study examined the effects of fruit and vegetable intake on the risk of stroke among middle-aged men, over twenty years of follow-up. The participants were 832 men, aged forty-five to sixty-five, who were free of cardio-vascular disease at the inception of the study (1966 to 1969). The diet of each subject as a baseline was assessed by a single twenty-four-hour recall. The estimated total number of servings per day of fruits and vegetables was the exposure variable for this analysis. The main outcome measured was the incidence of completed strokes and transient ischemic attacks.

During the twenty-year follow-up there were ninety-seven strokes, including seventy-three completed strokes and twenty-four transient ischemic attacks. Adjustment for body mass index, cigarette smoking, glucose intolerance, physical activity, blood pressure, serum cholesterol, and the intake of calories, alcohol, and fat did not materially change the results. After statistical analysis the authors concluded that increased intake of fruits and vegetables may well protect against the development of stroke in men.

Can the addition of vitamin C to the diet alter the incidence of stroke in elderly people? To determine this, British investigators did a twenty-year study of 730 men and women in England, Scotland, and Wales. At the outset the participants had no history or symptoms of stroke, cerebral artery sclerosis, or coronary heart disease.

The study found that mortality from stroke was highest in those participants with the lowest intake of vitamin C. Those participants with the highest intake of vitamin C had the lowest risk of stroke, after adjustment for age, sex, and established cardiovascular risk factors. The relationship between vitamin C intake and stroke was independent of social class and other dietary variables. A similar gradient in risk was present for plasma vitamin C concentrations. No similar relationship was found between vitamin C status and the risk of death from coronary heart disease. On the other hand, researchers from Northwestern University medical school who investigated 1,843 middle-aged men over a period of thirty years found only a modest decrease in the risk of stroke with a higher intake of beta-carotene and vitamin C.

A review of the medical literature undertaken by a research group in Cambridge, England, on the relationship of vitamin C intake to cardiovascular disease was somewhat consistent with the 1995 British study. The literature reviewers concluded that the evidence, although limited, is consistent with vitamin C supplementation having a protective effect against stroke. However, the evidence that vitamin C is protective against coronary heart disease is less compelling.

The effect of dietary flavonoids (diet supplements) on stroke was studied by a research group in the Netherlands. The researchers commented on the fact that many antioxidant preparations contain not only vitamin C but also flavonoids. They studied a group of 552 men aged fifty to sixty-nine years and followed them for fifteen years. Adjustments were made for confounding by age, systolic blood pressure, serum cholesterol, cigarette smoking, energy intake, and consumption of fish and alcohol.

Over the time of the study, forty-two cases of fatal or nonfatal stroke were documented. Dietary flavonoids (mainly quercetin) were inversely associated with the incidence of stroke. This was true even after adjustment for potential confounders, including antioxidant vitamins. In other words, certain dietary flavonoids seem to have a protective effect against stroke.

In February 1998, public health researchers from Taiwan studied the relationship between the concentrations of calcium and magnesium in drinking water and the risk of death from cerebrovascular disease. They examined 17,133 cases of cerebral vascular death from 1989 through 1993. These individuals were compared with people who had died from other causes

(17,133 controls), and levels of calcium and magnesium in drinking water of these persons were determined. The results of the study showed that there was a significant protective effect of magnesium intake from drinking water on the risk of cerebrovascular disease. However, this relationship was not true for calcium.

The relationship between the intake of ocean fish, like salmon or tuna, and the incidence of cardiovascular and cerebrovascular disease is unclear at the present time. However, it is clear that the intake of freshwater fish does not convey a protective effect. This was particularly true in a study from a public health institute in Finland. Freshwater lake fish tend to have an increased concentration of mercury in their bodies. These researchers presented data suggesting that a high intake of mercury was associated with an excess risk of death from cardiovascular disease.

A group of researchers from the University of Virginia school of medicine studied the effect of dietary calcium and milk consumption on the risk of nonhemorrhagic stroke in older middle-aged men. They concluded that an association between milk consumption and a reduced risk of stroke in older middle-aged men could not be explained by the intake of dietary calcium, even though there was evidence that dietary calcium was protective against hypertension. Since milk was often part of a diverse pattern of dietary intake, it was difficult to determine whether milk consumption had a direct role in reducing the risk of stroke. Their data did suggest that consumption of milk in older middle age is not harmful, and when combined with a balanced diet, weight control, and physical activity, reductions in the risk of stroke may occur.

The Centers for Disease Control and Prevention in Atlanta, Georgia, studied the level of serum folate and the risk for nonhemorrhagic stroke. They reviewed 2,006 individuals over thirteen years, and during that time ninety-eight nonhemorrhagic strokes occurred in their population. Using the appropriate statistical techniques and adjustments, they found that participants with a low serum concentration of folate were at a slightly increased risk for nonhemorrhagic stroke. It is my conclusion from this and other studies that dietary supplementation with folate and vitamin B-6 reduces homocysteine concentrations in the blood, and by this mechanism, there is a reduction in atherosclerotic vascular disease of both the heart and brain.

Reports on the effect of alcohol intake on the incidence of stroke have varied. A Japanese study in 1995 on 1,621 individuals came to the conclusion that among hypertensive individuals, heavy alcohol consumption leads to a significant increase in the risk of cerebral hemorrhage. These investigators suggested that there was a synergistic effect of alcohol and hypertension. They also suggested that light alcohol consumption reduced the risk of nonhemorrhagic strokes. In another study, the protective effects of alcohol intake on the incidence of stroke occurred only when the beverage was taken no more than once a day, for a total of five drinks a week. Increasing alcohol intake, it was found, increases the incidence of both hemorrhagic and nonhemorrhagic stroke. In fact, with increasing alcoholic intake, there is not only an increase in the incidence of cerebrovascular disease, but also of cardiovascular disease and coronary disease.

It has been suggested by some clinicians that red wine, by virtue of its relatively high concentration of polyphenols, is more protective against atherosclerosis than white wine. It has also been suggested that grape juice, enriched in one of these compounds, may share some of the properties of red wine. The test hypothesis was that these compounds would reduce atherosclerosis by reducing the enzyme thrombin induced platelet aggregation.

The researchers concluded from their studies that the active ingredients from grape juice (such as trans-resveratrol) are present in biologically significant quantities and in amounts that are likely to cause reduction in the risk of atherosclerosis. The failure of red wines (which have a twenty-fold excess of polyphenols over white wines) to show any advantage over white wines suggests that alcohol is the dominant anti-aggregation component in these beverages. Wine was more potent than grape juice in producing the anti-aggregation effect.

One of the most helpful investigations leading to a reduction in the incidence of strokes was carried out in London in 1997. It was a double-blind randomized trial of modest salt restriction in older people. Stroke is directly related to blood pressure. Treatment trials in older hypertensive individuals had shown a reduction in the incidence of strokes. However, the majority of strokes occur in normotensive individuals, that is, people with "normal" blood pressure, in whom no attempt is made to lower blood pressure. ("Normal" is defined as blood pressure that is less than 140 mm mercury systolic and 90 mm mercury diastolic.)

The investigators in this study compared the effects of modest salt restriction on blood pressure in forty-seven elderly hypertensive and normotensive people. Some interesting results came out of the two-month, double-blind, randomized placebo-controlled crossover study. With modest sodium restriction, a reduction in systolic blood pressure of 7.2 mm of mercury occurred. There was no significant difference in the blood pressure fall between eighteen normotensive and twenty-nine hypertensive participants. A modest reduction in salt intake leads to a fall in blood pressure in both normotensive and hypertensive older people similar to that in the outcome trials of antihypertensive medication. Since the majority of strokes in older people occur below the current definition of hypertension, these results have important implications for the prevention of stroke in the elderly.

We have known for some time that a decrease in saturated fat in the diet is associated with a decrease in the incidence of coronary artery disease. We also know from clinical experience that there is a distinct relationship between the incidence of heart attacks and strokes. It is not unusual for one to follow the other. Therefore, it was particularly confusing to get the report of the Framingham, Massachusetts, heart study, which showed that the risk of nonhemorrhagic stroke decreased when the quantity of total fat in the diet increased. It was even more confusing to find that the incidence of nonhemorrhagic stroke decreased with the increasing intake of saturated fat — but not with polyunsaturated fat. However, there was also a substantial decrease in the incidence of stroke with the increasing intake of monounsaturated fat.

A study from a department of epidemiology in Tokyo showed similar results. The Japanese researchers found that the relative risk for cerebral infarction was lowest in that segment of their population that ingested the highest level of total fat and saturated fatty acids. And the risk of cerebral infarction (nonhemorrhagic stroke) was highest in the people who took the greatest amount of polyunsaturated fatty acids in their diet.

However, an opposite effect was described by neurological researchers in Italy. They found that a low dietary intake of unsaturated fatty acids had been found in male patients with stroke as compared with controls. In their report, they cited a study in Australia that found a high consumption of meat associated with an increased risk of stroke. They presented a case control study, comparing the unsaturated and saturated fatty acid content of red cell membranes (which reflects the dietary intake of saturated and unsaturated fats) in eighty-nine patients with ischemic stroke and eighty-nine controls matched for age and sex. The stroke patients showed a lower level of unsaturated fatty acids as compared to the controls. These results confirmed a possible protective role for unsaturated fatty acids against vascular diseases. The researchers concluded that the preceding diet of patients with nonhemorrhagic stroke was deficient in unsaturated fatty acids.

Obviously, there is conflicting evidence regarding the relationship of the intake of dietary fats to the occurrence of nonhemorrhagic strokes. I believe that the safest dietary course involves the intake of monounsaturated fatty acids, such as those that occur in canola oil, olive oil, and even small amounts of peanut oil. I think it would be counterproductive to increase the saturated fat in your diet in the hope that it would reduce your chances of suffering a stroke. There is certainly enough evidence indicating that this kind of diet would increase your chance of having a heart attack. Why have either, especially if you can avoid them?

Finally, there is evidence from experimental studies that strokes in animals may be repaired by the implantation of fetal nerve cells. This technique has already been used to reverse the symptoms of patients with Parkinson's disease. Research on the development of stem cells, cloning, and other nuclear transplantation techniques is progressing rapidly. I have high hopes that this technique can eventually be used to repair the brain damage caused by strokes. Help from this technique is not presently available, but it will be in the near future.

Vital Memory Points to Remember

1. Multi-infarct dementia, which causes memory loss, is the result of tiny strokes that occur deep inside the brain.
2. Doctors sometimes confuse multi-infarct dementia with Alzheimer's disease.
3. Multi-infarct dementia is the second most common irreversible cause of memory loss and mental impairment.
4. Measures to prevent strokes include
   - following a low-fat diet (especially one restricted in saturated fats)
   - treating high blood pressure and avoiding low blood pressure
   - avoiding nicotine and tobacco
   - exercising moderately but regularly
   - avoiding excessive salt in the diet.
5. The effects of some major strokes can be reversed by prompt intravascular injections that dissolve blood clots.

19

Surgically Treatable Causes of Memory Loss

Subdural Hematomas

ANY OF US CAN get hit on the head hard enough to cause a blood clot pressing on the brain, which may produce memory problems. Blood clots that press on the brain, most frequently the variety known as subdural hematomas, are called the "great imitators" because the signs and symptoms they produce can imitate many neurological and psychiatric syndromes. If the blood clots are toward the front of the brain, they can produce apathy and attention deficits. If they are farther back, they can produce weakness or numbness. And if they grow to large size, they can produce all these symptoms. Moreover, because they shift the brain stem, they can cause decreased consciousness, paralysis, and a change in pupil size.

These blood clots are also classified as to whether they occur acutely and produce dramatic changes in the brain or whether, as frequently happens, they expand slowly over a period of days or weeks. They are then often accompanied by headaches and a rather unusual tenderness and sensitivity of the scalp. Even the chronic ones, if left unattended over six to eight weeks, can produce a major loss of intellectual function, including a loss of memory abilities.

Chronic Subdural Hematomas in the Elderly   Chronic subdural hematomas are more frequent in the elderly than in people in their twenties and thirties. This diagnosis is often missed in patients who are unsteady and especially prone to fall and hit their heads. Many patients who have chronic subdural hematomas don't even recall that they've had a previous head injury, so a diagnosis is made on other grounds.

Connie was a seventy-six-year-old retired travel agent. She had had several small strokes, but her condition had stabilized and she was able to walk around and largely take care of herself. About six months before I saw her she had been admitted to another hospital where evaluation of her brain function, including a CAT scan of her brain, had been made without showing any remarkable deviations from normal.

One morning Connie seemed to grow faint in the shower and was a little dizzy. Her daughter thought she might have suffered another small stroke and also noted that her mother's memory wasn't as good as it had been before this episode, and that her walking was not as facile. Her daughter called the doctor, who told her to get Connie back to the hospital for a workup. But because Connie had had a normal CAT scan six months before, the emergency room doctor felt that it was unnecessary to repeat the examination, and he sent her home again.

Over the next three or four days, Connie had a bit more difficulty walking. A psychiatrist who saw her said that her trouble in walking, what he called the "leaning tower of Pisa syndrome," was not unusual in persons taking the tranquilizer she was on.

Her daughter, however, was not satisfied with this answer. She called the attending doctor and again asked him to have another examination done. Since the original hospital refused to do further examinations she brought Connie to my office, where we found that she had some weakness, especially in one leg (accounting for the "leaning tower" when she walked) and a loss of recent memory. A CAT scan of the brain showed an enormous blood clot pressing the brain from one side to the other. The clot was subsequently removed, with a fair return of memory and other intellectual functions.

It was a good thing Connie's daughter was so persistent. The blood clot had displaced brain tissue to the extent that Connie's life would have been in danger, or at least irreversible brain damage threatened, if diagnosis and treatment had been further delayed.

Occasionally small subdural hematomas will clear up without surgical drainage — but don't bank on it. Some patients treated conservatively by neurological physicians have succumbed to sudden shifts in pressure within their skulls. Except with very small hematomas, I believe that surgical evacuation is the wisest course in almost every case.

Ruling Out Subdural Hematomas as a Cause of Memory Loss   In any case of memory loss one should consider subdural hematoma as a possible cause that must be ruled out with a CAT scan or magnetic resonance imaging of the brain. This was especially true in the case of Elmer, a forty-nine-year-old shoe salesman admitted with a primary diagnosis of depression and memory loss to a nearby mental hospital. He was lucky that an astute neurologist was asked to consult on his case. Before allowing Elmer's psychiatrist to go further with medications or electroshock treatment, the neurologist asked for a CAT scan, which showed a large subdural hematoma that had produced a dangerous shift in brain structures.

The treatment of this man's problem by removing the hematoma was so gratifying, and the reversal of symptoms so prompt, that everyone was pleased — the psychiatrist, for discharging his patient as cured; the neurologist, for discovering the problem; but most of all the patient, who regained memory and mental functions after being misdiagnosed as having a severe, intractable depression.

Subdural hematoma is a great imitator of brain disability and disease, and even many psychiatric syndromes. In psychiatric and neurological cases in which the diagnosis is in doubt, a CAT or MRI scan is simple to do and will rule out this completely treatable problem.

Brain Tumors

What would you think if your doctor told you that the cause of your memory loss was a brain tumor? First and foremost, you need not panic. Many brain tumors are benign, and with modern surgical techniques they can be cured. Second, don't imagine that your doctor is likely to find that your symptoms are caused by a brain tumor. Unlike what you may have been led to believe by watching television soap operas or reading sensational tabloids, brain tumors are relatively uncommon in our population, constituting about 2 percent of all the tumors found in humans.

What you must keep in mind is that most brain tumors are treatable and many are curable, together with their symptom of memory loss if it occurs. Brain tumors must be diagnosed early, however; if left untreated, the increased pressure within the head which they generate will impair not only memory but many other brain functions. They interfere with normal brain function either by just the mass effect of the tumor itself, or by obstructing the flow of spinal fluid, causing a backup and expansion of the fluid spaces in the brain in the condition called hydrocephalus. The increased pressure is relayed into the backs of the eyeballs, where the optic nerve heads are located, and these structures tend to swell, causing a loss of vision.

Brain tumors, of course, damage brain tissue locally by direct pressure on the tissue, and there is often additional damage to the surrounding brain because of swelling or edema caused by the advancing tumor itself. A tumor can also interfere with the blood supply to the brain, and, of course, it can irritate the brain tissue around it to produce epileptic seizures.

How Brain Tumors Affect Memory Even when a brain tumor doesn't invade memory pathways, it may still impede mental processes and recent memory because of increased pressure and its effects within the head. That's what happened to Andy, a fifty-two-year-old carpet cleansing manager, before he entered the hospital. About nine months prior to when I saw him he had complained to his physicians of severe pain in his head, which was worse when he put his head forward or changed its position suddenly. Shortly afterward his business associates noted that he was not as sharp in his business dealings or as responsible as he had been. The company he worked for started to lose money because of the decisions Andy made, and in a desperate effort to recoup some of it for them, Andy made choices that only made matters worse.

When I saw him, Andy walked with a wide-based gait and was unsteady on his feet. His optic nerve heads were swollen, indicating that he had increased pressure in his brain, and he had a major loss of intellectual function and particular difficulty with recent memory.

Special x-ray tests showed that he had a tumor in the back part of his brain, which obstructed the flow of spinal fluid, producing hydrocephalus. Subsequently the mass was completely removed by surgery, and he had a dramatic recovery. The increased pressure in his head subsided completely and his intellectual ability returned, with vast improvement of his recent memory. Unfortunately, the return of his mental abilities didn't happen in time to save his job. With his previous contacts and his regained health, however, he found new employment and now has a good chance to become successful again in the commercial marketplace.

Other Types of Brain Tumors That Affect Memory   The type of tumor Andy had, a glioma, is the most common variety. Other kinds can bring about similar but different symptoms. A slow-growing tumor in the front part of the brain (a meningioma) can produce gradual deterioration in intellectual abilities and memory which may escape notice for a number of years. That was the situation in the case of Helga, a forty-seven-year-old business executive who owned an exclusive and profitable modeling agency and who also manufactured and distributed cosmetics. I was asked to see her after she had been charged by the Internal Revenue Service with evading $2.3 million in taxes over a three-year period.

Her defense at first didn't seem very good. She claimed not to have any memory of conferences with her lawyers or with IRS agents, conferences that were critical to the case against her. Helga was unlike the typical person charged with tax evasion, however. Well after the IRS investigation of her finances started, she began to have difficulty with her vision, and it was noticed that her optic nerve head was swollen and she had increased pressure in her brain. CAT scans and magnetic resonance images showed a slow-growing tumor in the front part of her brain which was as big as a tangerine. It threatened her life and was promptly removed. But even after surgery her personality did not revert to normal, although her brain function, including recent memory, gradually improved.

The tumor had not only compressed part of her brain but also obstructed its blood supply. The resultant scarring in the area generated occasional epileptic seizures. Because the tumor had been in the frontal rather than the temporal lobes, it didn't directly interfere with the memory circuits. It did, however, through interrupting frontal lobe function, produce apathy, a symptom hard to distinguish from severe depression in

240

its effects on concentration and attention. Thus the tumor disturbed the acquisition of new memories, and it slowed Helga's ability to retrieve memories from her memory bank.

The removal of Helga's brain tumor improved her memory abilities, but they were still intermittently and unpredictably disrupted by the localized epileptic seizures at the site where the brain tumor had been. Subsequently her memory was further improved by the administration of antiseizure drugs. As for her troubles with the IRS, the government had a rather weak case against her, and the case was settled in her favor. No one with a sizable tumor like Helga's should be convicted of tax evasion.

Once a tumor is suspected, diagnosis can be readily made with imaging techniques like CAT and MRI scans. Making such a diagnosis early is crucial because early treatment, whether by surgical excision or sometimes radiation therapy, not only improves the chances that a complete cure will be effected but can also relieve symptoms and reverse memory loss.

Hydrocephalus

Guess what Beethoven and Amenhotep IV, the pharaoh who introduced the worship of a single god in Egypt, had in common. All right, you give up? Both suffered the condition known as arrested hydrocephalus, a clinical problem that, in its controlled state, is compatible with great mental ability. Progressive hydrocephalus, however, whether caused by an obstruction such as a brain tumor or a constriction of the outflow ducts, will produce increased pressure within the skull and a significant decrease in intellectual and memory functions.

Elderly people tend to get a kind of hydrocephalus or accumulation of excess spinal fluid, with dilatation of the fluid-filled spaces, or ventricles, in the brain, without having increased pressure inside the head. This condition, called normal-pressure hydrocephalus, results from lowered brain elasticity, which allows any temporary increase in pressure in the ventricles to balloon them out. The effects on brain function — including loss of memory, incontinence, and especially difficulty walking — are great, even though the pressure inside the head remains normal.

To illustrate, I'd like to relate the case of Martha, seventy-two, who was a hard-working short-order cook and waitress who had successively helped support two alcoholic husbands, whom she divorced, and another who died of a heart attack. Martha had a long history of manic-depressive disease and was hospitalized on several occasions for many months. When I saw her she complained of "wicked" headaches and had severe difficulty walking. In fact, she couldn't walk without the aid of a three-pronged cane, and even then she seemed to stagger from one side of the hall to the other. The nurse who accompanied her said that, in addition, her memory was gone; she couldn't remember anything. "She lives from one minute to the next. I have to dress her and feed her," the nurse said.

A CAT scan of Martha's brain showed hugely dilated ventricles, way out of proportion to the shrinkage in the rest of her brain. Now hydrocephalus can be treated by an operation that shunts the spinal fluid through a one-way valve into the abdominal cavity, or even into the heart. But first radioactive tests need to be done to trace the flow of spinal fluid and confirm the diagnosis. I find one of the more reliable predictive indicators of successful surgical treatment to be repeated spinal punctures, with the removal of spinal fluid. If the removal of spinal fluid improves memory and especially walking, the shunting procedure has a high chance of being effective. Because preliminary removal of spinal fluid gave her temporary relief from her symptoms on several occasions, Martha had surgery, which proved to be successful.

The shunting procedure in older patients with hydrocephalus has lost popularity among some physicians because dementia and memory loss are not reversed in a few patients. This result is not because the operation doesn't remove the excess spinal fluid; it is rather that these patients actually have two diseases: hydrocephalus and Alzheimer's disease or Binswanger's disease (border zone infarcts), which also allows the ventricles to dilate. Of course, surgical treatment is not effective for either of the latter conditions. Even in Alzheimer's patients with hydrocephalus, however, improvement in walking is often noted.

Hydrocephalus can be ruled out with a CAT scan or magnetic resonance imaging, and thus it will be picked up on the usual battery of tests given to patients who have memory loss or other deterioration in their mental abilities. It is good to keep in mind that hydrocephalus can also be a consequence of brain injury or brain hemorrhage, and that mental deterioration or persistent memory loss in patients demands proper imaging of the brain to rule out this treatable and reversible problem.

Hydrocephalus and Aggressive Behavior Kenneth, an eighty-two-year-old candy store owner, was a kindly widower who spent much of his time serving the young customers who came to his shop on their way home from school. One spring afternoon a child who had visited his store stepped off the sidewalk in front of a car, and Kenneth rushed into the street, pushed the child out of the way, and was himself hit by the motorist, who had vainly tried to stop. Kenneth was unconscious for a while and was sent to a neighborhood hospital, where he was found to have blood in his spinal fluid. He recovered over a period of four or five days, and after a ten-day period he was sent to stay with his son and daughter-in-law.

Kenneth's behavior became more unusual as the weeks passed. Unlike most hydrocephalic patients, who become sleepy and lethargic, Kenneth became quite aggressive. He also had memory loss and occasional incontinence. One morning while he was shaving himself with a straight razor he whipped it around and threatened his daughter-in-law, saying, "I'm going to cut your head off." She ran screaming from the apartment.

When Kenneth was brought into the hospital he had very pronounced hydrocephalus, which was treated by the shunting procedure. When he awoke from surgery he told the female resident who was taking care of him, "Kiss me, sweetie, or I'll punch you in the nose." Over the next several days, however, he improved remarkably, and his aggressive tendencies disappeared. Kenneth's memory also improved, and his walking was quite stable.

Proper Diagnosis Cases like Kenneth's are unusual because, as noted above, most people with this disorder experience lethargy along with other symptoms such as recent-memory loss, trouble walking and a tendency to fall, and incontinence. The lesson to remember as far as hydrocephalus is concerned is the same one conveyed in the previous sections on subdural hematomas and brain tumors: when the diagnosis is in doubt, include a CAT scan or magnetic resonance imaging in the patient's evaluation. These techniques allow us not only to diagnose but to visualize in detail well over 90 percent of all the surgically treatable problems of the brain discussed in this chapter. I also feel strongly that the use of these diagnostic tools should be considered for persons with unexplained psychiatric symptoms, including personality changes, as well as for patients with obvious brain disease.

Vital Memory Points to Remember
1. Subdural hematomas are blood clots that press on the brain, whose effects can imitate many different neurological and psychiatric syndromes.

2. Brain tumors often interfere with mental processes and recent memory because of increased pressure within the head.
3. Prompt diagnosis of these problems by CAT scan or magnetic resonance imaging allows early treatment to be undertaken and therefore improves outcomes.

20

Degenerative Brain Disease and Memory Loss

THE DEGENERATIVE BRAIN DISORDERS are those characterized by a loss of brain tissue and corresponding mental function. Some of these disorders, such as multiple sclerosis, have a sputtering course; they flare up for a while, then a period of months or even years may ensue in which there are no symptoms. Others, like Parkinson's disease, progress slowly but steadily, causing a loss of tissue and a deficiency of neurotransmitters deep in the brain. Still others, like Alzheimer's, have a more rapid course, producing a loss of tissue in the cortex, the surface of the brain.

In this chapter I concentrate on Alzheimer's, which we have also touched on earlier in this book, because it is the most frequent cause of irreversible memory loss in the elderly. The onset of this disease may vary, but memory problems — particularly loss of recent memory — are always prominent. Some people with the disease have degeneration in the speech areas of the brain, making it difficult for them to name objects. Tissue degeneration in others disturbs their orientation — for example, their ability to find their destination in a car or even on foot. Whatever the pattern of brain loss, it progresses until all of the above symptoms of brain loss are prominent. The patterns themselves are not invariable, however, and it is likely that the name "Alzheimer's" describes more than one degenerative brain disease.

The words *Alzheimer's disease* are among the most feared in the vocabularies of persons over the age of forty-five because they raise the specter of irreversible and devastating memory loss and mental helplessness. People seem to feel that there is a certain inevitability about the disease, and many (including some doctors) equate it with aging or senility.

Myths About Alzheimer's Disease

To begin this discussion of Alzheimer's disease, I'd like to dispel some myths about it. First, normal aging does not produce senility or Alzheimer's. That is a well-established medical fact. Second, although Alzheimer's is a diagnosis of exclusion, only to be confirmed by the characteristic changes in the brain seen at post-mortem examination, its clinical picture may represent more than one disease with different causes and, eventually, quite different treatments. Third, although some people have a genetic predisposition to develop Alzheimer's disease, which is perhaps more strongly manifested in victims who get the disorder before the age of fifty-five, inheritance doesn't explain all the factors that lead to the clinical expression of the disease.

Causes of Alzheimer's Disease

There are lots of theories about what causes Alzheimer's. Early in 1991, Dr. John Hardy of St. Mary's Hospital in London announced that he and his colleagues had discovered at least one of the genes that cause Alzheimer's. According to the researchers, a mutation occurs in the gene which directs cells to produce a protein called beta amyloid, a component of nerve cells. It is this protein that is thought to be responsible for the disease. This research on the role of beta amyloid has been amplified by work at Duke University and Massachusetts

General Hospital. However, the final resolution of this multi-factorial problem has not yet been reached.

Slow viral infections of the brain have been raised as a possible inciting factor. Also, the ingestion of certain metals, such as aluminum, has been under investigation (I must add without much in the way of convincing evidence). Decreased lecithin or choline has been put forward as a cause of the loss of cells in the cholinergic circuit related to the memory process. The overaccumulation of organic compounds related to glutamate (glutamic acid), which kills nerve cells by producing an excess amount of calcium around them, has been suggested as a mechanism in various degenerative brain diseases. Other proposed factors include chronic alcohol abuse with repeated head injury and even poor intellectual attainment.

There has been some genetic linking as a causal factor for Alzheimer's to patients who have a very early onset, especially those patients with Down's syndrome. But there are also some patients with late-onset Alzheimer's who may also have a genetic factor.

Late-onset Alzheimer's disease does show familial clustering but does not show a clear mode of inheritance. The only genetic determinant universally accepted as an important risk factor for late-onset Alzheimer's disease is what is known as the apolipoprotein-E locus on chromosome 19. (A lipoprotein is a protein molecule that binds lipids together so that they can be carried throughout the bloodstream, since lipids cannot be dissolved in the blood. Without getting too technical, the apo form is simply one type of lipoprotein.)

Scientists have found that a certain amount of familial clustering in late-onset Alzheimer's disease is accounted for by this genetic factor. However, the apolipoprotein connection appears to account for, at most, about half the genetic risk of developing the disease. Thus, other genes or risk factors must be involved, and they are, at present, unknown.

248

Diagnosis of Alzheimer's Disease

Researchers in a number of centers are working on ways to enable us to make a positive diagnosis of Alzheimer's disease before death. One of the more promising leads is the discovery of a protein in the brain which is present in about 85 percent of people who have the diagnosis of Alzheimer's confirmed at post-mortem examination. This substance may be present in the spinal fluid as well, and thus a positive diagnosis might be possible by identifying this protein in specimens of spinal fluid obtained by lumbar puncture.

I personally believe that it is a mistake to concentrate on early diagnosis of Alzheimer's disease before there is effective treatment. Once the diagnosis of Alzheimer's disease is established, too many physicians give up any attempt to search out other treatable problems that might be making the Alzheimer's patient worse, and the patient is prematurely sent to a nursing home. Tests should therefore be used only in the end stages of the disease, and in the meantime we should continue to look for conditions (even in suspected Alzheimer's cases) that are treatable and reversible. The role of the much-publicized abnormal protein in Alzheimer's should not be underestimated, however, since it may well be the key to determining the causal mechanisms in many cases of the disease, and in turn to discovering effective treatment and prevention strategies.

Radioactive PET and SPECT (single photon emission computerized tomography) scans detect abnormally reduced metabolism in certain areas of the brain in Alzheimer's patients. But caution is necessary: other degenerative diseases that at post-mortem prove not to be Alzheimer's can have a similar radioactive scan pattern. Also, brain mapping using quantitative brain wave recordings shows slower activity in Alzheimer's patients than in depressed patients.

Dealing with Alzheimer's

Most patients with Alzheimer's disease don't complain about memory loss or their failing mental abilities because the critical faculty in the brain which allows them to monitor their own behavior is often lost quite early in the course of the illness. That is not to say that some patients with Alzheimer's are not quite depressed and fearful about what's happening to them, but this is usually not the case. Most people who come into my office with detailed complaints about their loss of memory are suffering from one of the reversible disorders, most commonly depression.

Another misconception about Alzheimer's is that it only occurs after the age of fifty. The frequency of its occurrence does increase after fifty, and even more after eighty, but it's a disorder that can occur at any age. Especially in children with Down's syndrome, Alzheimer's disease can manifest itself as early as age fifteen or sixteen.

I was recently challenged by an official at the National Institute of Aging when I said that even skillful neurologists are mistaken in their diagnosis of Alzheimer's disease in 12 to 20 percent of cases. My comment was based on the results of a study done at the University of Toronto's Sunnybrook Medical Center which reviewed post-mortem examinations of the brains of patients who, when they were alive, had been diagnosed by more than one doctor as having Alzheimer's disease. More than 14 percent of these patients had actually had a problem other than Alzheimer's.

The doctor who questioned my information said that recent studies using magnetic resonance imaging as well as new psychological research brought the error rate down to between 5 and 10 percent. Nevertheless, I maintain that he was overly optimistic and that the brains of many patients with the symptoms of Alzheimer's still do not, at post-mortem examinations, display the typical characteristics of the disease. In fact, some post-mortems have revealed the signs of Alzheimer's disease in patients who had had none of the symptoms. All this means is that there is a good deal of uncertainty about the diagnosis even among very experienced neurologists at major medical centers. If we were to consider the diagnosis of this disorder in general medical practice, we would have a much higher error rate, probably approaching 30 percent.

Reversible Complications in Alzheimer's Patients

The progression of Alzheimer's disease from slight to very severe dementia varies from individual to individual. Even when the disease is properly diagnosed, it can be still complicated by a number of other factors which make the symptoms much worse. Disorders like depression, brain poisoning with alcohol or prescription drugs, malnutrition, and even sensory monotony can nudge a patient who would be marginally self-sufficient into a state of complete dependence. That's why it's so important to check for treatable disorders even in patients who do have Alzheimer's. The correction of treatable problems can improve patients' clinical pictures enough so that they will be able to function independently for a much longer period of time than they would if these problems were neglected. These additional causes of memory loss are more likely to occur in the nursing home setting, where sensory deprivation, depression, and especially brain poisoning with prescription drugs are all too common.

Hereditary Diseases

Almost any degenerative brain disease may progress to the point that loss of memory and of intellectual function occurs, although mental impairment is much less common in the early stages of multiple sclerosis and Parkinson's disease. The time course varies greatly in the different disorders. Memory loss and mental deterioration are, of course, the hallmarks

251

of Alzheimer's from the onset of the syndrome. By contrast, people with multiple sclerosis can remain static for decades, with no sign of mental deterioration or memory loss, whereas Parkinson's disease usually advances more quickly.

Another degenerative brain disease similar to Alzheimer's is called degenerative dementia (or dementia with Lewy bodies). This disease has become increasingly well recognized in the last twenty years. Of course, the two most common degenerative brain diseases in older adults are still Alzheimer's disease and Parkinson's disease. While Alzheimer's disease begins with memory and other intellectual losses, Parkinson's disease is primarily a motor disease characterized by a pill-rolling tremor at rest, muscular rigidity, and difficulty in initiating movements. The onset of dementia occurs much later in the course of the illness.

Pathological examinations on post-mortem specimens of the brain in some patients with a degenerative dementia with Lewy bodies have shown certain similarities to the brains of those having pure Parkinson's disease. It is estimated that degenerative dementia, sometimes masquerading as Alzheimer's, or as an unusual form of Parkinson's, may account for as many as one-fourth of all people with some form of dementia. The initial symptoms of this disease include a loss of memory function along with motor disorders and confusional states. There are more psychiatric symptoms in this disease, with such things as visual hallucinations occurring in 60 to 80 percent of the patients, than in Parkinson's disease, or even in most cases of Alzheimer's disease.

Certain people with degenerative dementia may also have an action tremor of their limbs and some rigidity of their trunk. The motor signs of the disease are not as severe as they are in Parkinson's. However, confusion and visual hallucinations are much more common in this disorder than in Parkinson's.

The recognition of this disorder points out the fact that our attempts at accurate diagnosis, explanation of the origins of dementing illnesses, and the possible prevention of such illnesses are still in an early stage of evolution. This entire area of brain research will assume increasing importance as more and more people reach an advanced age and become susceptible to these disorders. This kind of brain research will require an enormous increase in the level of federal financial support.

Treatment

The fact that a disease is hereditary, as some cases of Alzheimer's may well be, does not mean that it is untreatable. Wilson's disease, for example, an inherited disorder causing degeneration of the inner parts of the brain and portions of the liver, may start as early as the second decade of life with a tremor of the limbs and head, slowness of movement, abnormal behavior, and finally loss of intellectual function, with loss of memory among other symptoms. Medical researchers have found that the genetic deficiency that causes Wilson's disease works by producing abnormally large deposits of copper, especially in the liver and brain. When these concentrations are reduced the symptoms of the disease can often be reversed, and many patients are brought back to normal brain function. Just as we have been able to treat the inherited brain defect that produces Wilson's disease, within the next ten to fifteen years we will be able to do the same for those patients who have inherited Alzheimer's disease.

One of the most difficult messages to deliver to families in which a member is stricken with an incurable degenerative brain disease is the message that they must not give up hope. Even if we don't now have an effective treatment for Alzheimer's disease, extensive research is being done which may lead to its eventual prevention and cure. And even when brain tissue has been lost, we may in the future be able to replace it with fetal nerve cell transplants.

In the meantime, and to reiterate my point on the treatment

of patients with Alzheimer's disease, we must make every effort to diagnose other conditions that may make the symptoms of Alzheimer's, especially its attendant memory loss, worse than they need to be, and to treat those problems that are reversible promptly. Moreover, I want to stress to caregivers the importance of providing Alzheimer's victims every memory aid available. Such aids include establishing a firm and consistent routine to keep patients in one location, prominently displaying dates and times in large block letters near patients' beds or chairs, and making rooms they use easily accessible so that they can carry on their usual routines without getting lost. For example, ensure that they can get to the bathroom by themselves, and guard against their being able to lock themselves in or out. Also, doorways leading outside or to other potentially dangerous areas should be locked to prevent wandering in strange and difficult places.

Finally, caregivers to persons with Alzheimer's must learn to provide the level of assistance that is needed without smothering the abilities that patients still have for independent action. This means assessing their individual abilities and offering only the amount of help necessary for safety. It also means exercising patience in allowing patients to express their remaining talents, even if these are much reduced in quality, spontaneity, and speed. It means supporting them when they are frustrated and encouraging them when they falter. It means not getting angry when they make mistakes and never taking their anger or hostility seriously.

From this catalogue you can see how difficult it is to be a caregiver to an Alzheimer's patient. Imagine how much more difficult it would be for a member of the family to assume the role. Unlike a nurse who steps into the caregiving function from outside, family members can't forget how their loved one was before, and they can't stop mentally comparing the patient's present invalidism with past prowess.

It is gratifying, nevertheless, to hear the story of a man who was devotedly cared for by his sister, who kept him in the home he'd lived in for more than forty-five years. For fifteen years after he became ill with Alzheimer's disease, his sister guided him, with increasing assistance as time went on, in an unvarying routine, including seeing the same people at the same time each day. Even though he progressively lost brain tissue, he was able to live and function for a much longer period than most Alzheimer's victims.

Obviously, Alzheimer's disease varies in its intensity and rate of progression from person to person. We must therefore fit the treatment and the circumstances to each individual and not push patients prematurely into institutions that will make their intellectual and memory deficits worse. Let me emphasize that there *are* some people whose brain disease has advanced to such an extent that they are helpless. Unless they are well-to-do and can afford round-the-clock nursing care, institutionalization is the only alternative available to them. My plea is that institutionalization not occur until absolutely necessary. I have seen too many lives wasted that could otherwise have been productive in the so-called golden years, had complete diagnosis and correct treatment been carried out.

When this book was first published, there were no proven effective treatments for Alzheimer's disease. The situation has now changed. There are still no cures for Alzheimer's disease, but there are treatments that seem to slow down the progression of the disease.

Central cholinergic neurotransmission plays an important role in the formation of memory and new learning. The neurotransmitter acetylcholine is pivotal in this function. Since acetylcholine in the hippocampus (an important center in the brain for the formation of new memories) is reduced in Alzheimer's disease, it was thought that the memory deficit in Alzheimer's patients could be improved by substantially increasing the amount of choline in the brain. Although increasing choline in the brain does have beneficial effects as far as certain kinds of memory function is concerned, these effects are only seen in normal individuals. The beneficial effects do not seem to occur in people with Alzheimer's.

Another treatment strategy that has been tried was to inhibit the enzymes called cholinesterases, which react chemically with acetylcholine at nerve synapses. When the cholinesterases were inhibited, the quantity of acetylcholine at the synapses dramatically increased. The class of drugs that inhibit the cholinesterases are called cholinesterase inhibitors. A number of these drugs were tried in experimental animals and in human studies, some of which seem to produce a slight positive effect. The first of these drugs to show promise in humans was a drug called tacrine.

This drug was used in five double-blind, placebo-controlled multi-center trials, in more than 2,000 patients with uncomplicated mild to moderate Alzheimer's disease. Some of these trials showed that patients being treated with tacrine had a statistically significant improvement in memory function as contrasted with controls.

One-fifth of the patients were unable to tolerate this drug because of gastrointestinal distress. In higher doses, the drug was reversibly toxic to the liver in about one-half of the patients. Liver function tests began to be abnormal after six weeks of treatment. Most of these abnormalities were reversible when the drug was discontinued.

Donepezil (also called Aricept) is another more recently discovered cholinesterase inhibitor. It is a piperidine-based, reversible acetylcholine esterase inhibitor that has significantly greater selectivity for acetylcholine esterase than does tacrine. Also, compared to tacrine, it is longer lasting and is not as toxic. Still, like tacrine, it only slows down the pace of memory loss and other intellectual symptoms. It is not a cure for Alzheimer's disease.

Selegiline (deprenyl), an inhibitor drug, and alpha-tocopherol (vitamin E) have been used separately and in combination for the treatment of mental deterioration in people with Alzheimer's disease. In a randomized study, it was found that both of these drugs did delay functional deterioration, particularly with regard to the need for institutionalization. It was concluded that these agents were useful in people with a moderate dementia.

It should be noted that deprenyl, but not alpha-tocopherol, also significantly delayed the need for the use of potent medications, like levodopa, in people with Parkinson's disease. The benefit, however, was not sustained during long-term follow-up. Investigators have concluded that the symptomatic delay was probably not due to a slowing down of the underlying degenerative process in the brain. In a similar fashion, the use of these two drugs, deprenyl and tocopherol, while they slowed down the progression of some symptoms in Alzheimer's patients, probably did not affect the underlying degenerative process in the brain.

Nonsteroidal anti-inflammatory drugs, including aspirin, seem to have an effect in slowing down the progression and delaying the onset of Alzheimer's disease. In 1997, a longitudinal study was carried out by the department of epidemiology at Johns Hopkins School of Public Health. There it was found that the relative risk for the onset of Alzheimer's disease decreased with the increasing duration of nonsteroidal anti-inflammatory drug use. The greatest benefit timewise from this use was two years. After two years, the continued use of nonsteroidal anti-inflammatory drugs did not give added protection against Alzheimer's.

It has also been hypothesized that the use of estrogen replacement therapy in women reduces the risk of contracting Alzheimer's disease. A number of estrogenic properties support the biological credibility of this hypothesis. Certainly, we know that estrogen interacts with neurotransmitter systems that appear relevant to Alzheimer's disease.

Clinical studies of post-menopausal women suggest beneficial estrogen effects on specific cognitive skills, including certain aspects of memory. Small preliminary trials of estrogen replacement in women with Alzheimer's disease tend to support claims of clinical benefit. However, definitive double-blind, placebo-controlled longitudinal studies using matched controls have not yet been accomplished. So, for now, the issue of estrogen effectiveness in lowering a woman's risk for Alzheimer's disease remains unsettled.

Studies on the effect of a new agent, galantamine, were presented at the sixth international conference on Alzheimer's disease held in July 1998 in Amsterdam. Research indicates that this drug has a dual mechanism of action. On one hand, it is an acetylcholine esterase inhibitor. However, unlike other agents, galantamine also appears to act on the brain's nicotinic receptors; the modulation of these receptors could lead to the release of even more acetylcholine at the synapse.

In a double-blind placebo-controlled study in a U.S. trial, 636 people with mild to moderate Alzheimer's disease were enrolled. Four hundred twenty-three individuals were assigned to receive galantamine twice a day for six months, and 213 took placebos. Sixty-two percent of the patients were women, and the mean age of participants was seventy-five. Study participants were tested using the cognitive portion of the Alzheimer's disease assessment scale, which is commonly used to assess memory and learning skills such as word recall and recognition, ability to remember test instructions, and accuracy in naming objects and figures.

Among those who completed the study, those who took galantamine achieved memory scores that were an average of 3.7 to 3.8 points higher than individuals who received the placebo. Participants taking the placebo had a decline in their memory scores by 2 points over the course of the study. However, participants taking galantamine had an average improvement of 1.7 points over their beginning (baseline) score.

Improvements in those taking galantamine began to be apparent as soon as one week after reaching the target dose of the medicine. Adverse effects included nausea and other gastrointestinal side effects. However, these adverse effects usually were transient, often subsiding after one week on the medication.

It is obviously too early to draw definite conclusions about the usefulness of galantamine in the treatment of Alzheimer's disease, in spite of the early encouraging results. However, it is intriguing to note the effects of this drug on nicotinic receptors of the brain, which may partially explain the increased beneficial effects of this drug. This observation goes along with another recent study showing the delayed onset of Alzheimer's disease in post-menopausal women who not only took estrogen replacement therapy but also smoked cigarettes.

Vital Memory Points to Remember

1. Normal aging does not produce senility or Alzheimer's disease.
2. Alzheimer's, as a specific variety of dementia, is a diagnosis of exclusion which is usually only positively confirmed at post-mortem.
3. Genetics does not explain all the factors that lead to Alzheimer's. Do not think that just because one of your parents has Alzheimer's you are destined to get it.
4. A diagnosis of Alzheimer's disease does not necessarily mean that the patient is incompetent. I have seen Alzheimer's patients who, while disabled in one sphere, were competent in another — finance, say, or ornamental gardening. The degree of incompetence depends on the extent of tissue loss in the cortex of the brain in each patient.
5. Treatable causes of dementia may be present in Alzheimer's patients, and these conditions may make memory loss much worse than it needs to be. These disorders should be diagnosed and treated promptly.
6. Memory aids, a predictable routine, and intelligent patient monitoring are the essence of effective management

of Alzheimer's patients. Patients should be given enough independence to express their abilities and enough supervision to compensate for their deficits. The level of freedom has to be determined for each individual.

7. Advances in diagnostic methods offer hope that not only successful treatments for the symptoms of Alzheimer's but also techniques for preventing its progression will be developed.

Hope for the Future

21

Prevention: What You Can Do to Avoid Memory Loss

OVER THE LAST YEAR I've traveled through much of the eastern part of the United States, and I've had the chance to be on radio talk shows broadcast to the whole nation. The questions and concerns voiced from Alaska, California, and Oklahoma are much the same as those from New York, Pennsylvania, and Florida. Everyone wants to know what can be done to prevent a decline in memory and other intellectual functions and prolong useful life. I would like to review with you some of the questions I've been asked about memory loss and what treatments might reverse it, as well as about preventing memory loss and intellectual deterioration.

Preventing Memory Loss Associated with Alzheimer's

The question I hear most often is, "How can I prevent memory loss and keep from getting Alzheimer's disease?" At the present time we don't know precisely what causes Alzheimer's disease, and this knowledge is necessary for prevention. We think there may be an inherited predisposition in some cases, probably a minority of the cases. And this predisposition is more pronounced in persons who are afflicted with the disease before the age of fifty-five.

Statistical studies reviewed and reported by A. S. Henderson, a researcher in social psychiatry from the Australian National University in Canberra, report that the number of people showing clinical signs and symptoms of Alzheimer's disease increases consistently with age. He concluded that the process underlying the dementia that characterizes Alzheimer's becomes more intense with age. The peculiar thing about these statistics, however, is that the increase in the incidence of Alzheimer's disease with age stops abruptly at age ninety, when it begins to go down. We thus know that aging in itself is not a cause of the disease.

It has also been reported that more women than men have Alzheimer's, and that more men than women have multi-infarct dementia (small strokes). However, this observation may be biased because, since women live longer than men, there are more women in the older age groups that have a greater incidence of Alzheimer's disease.

It's also interesting to note that studies have been undertaken to differentiate the vulnerability of individuals to Alzheimer's disease on the basis of their social class and education. Several studies found the incidence of Alzheimer's disease among the well educated to be thirty times less than it is among the poorly educated. Because they are controversial, studies such as these have been criticized as being biased. In my opinion, the results are certainly astonishing, and there is no biological explanation for them. Furthermore, they don't square with my own experience, which is that well-to-do, highly educated people appear to get Alzheimer's disease as often as anyone else.

Correlates with Alzheimer's disease are a history of blood transfusion, a previous diagnosis of clinical depression, and a history of herpes zoster, a viral disease commonly known as shingles. Some researchers investigating the disease have also noted an association between primary dementia, or loss of intellectual function, and a past history of diabetes, physical inactivity, heart disease (particularly heart failure), and constipation. Alzheimer's disease and multi-infarct dementia occur together much more often than just by chance. It may be that the multiple small cerebral infarcts accelerate the clinical course — that is, increase the loss of memory and other intellectual functions which occurs in Alzheimer's.

Head injuries too have been implicated as a co-factor with Alzheimer's disease in two studies that found some statistical correlations between the two phenomena. Six other studies have failed to find the correlation, however, and in two others the correlation was not significant.

What risk factors are associated with Alzheimer's? Dr. J. Mortimer of the University of Minnesota has suggested that a family history of dementia is the most frequent risk factor, and prior head trauma the second most common factor. Other risk factors that have been suggested, without much evidence, include the use of antiperspirants containing aluminum, since increased levels of aluminum are among the pathological changes in the brains of Alzheimer's patients.

The possible role of aluminum in Alzheimer's disease has been widely publicized, causing a measure of hysteria in various communities in this country. In one case that I know about, the publicity caused an elderly woman to take drastic measures. Angelina, an eighty-six-year-old widow, was a meticulous housekeeper who collected bone china, dishes, and fine cooking utensils. Among other things, she had a collection of exquisite aluminum cookware and teapots. Angelina read somewhere about the theoretical connection between aluminum and Alzheimer's disease and how it afflicted people over the age of seventy-five. She immediately called her daughter to come over and dispose of every fine piece of aluminum in her collection.

What Angelina and many other people don't understand is that processes in the body reduce the amount of aluminum absorbed, particularly from the gastrointestinal tract. Also, many people don't realize that a number of commonly ingested antacids contain aluminum. Moreover, all of us take in a certain amount of aluminum in our food. If the metal did have a significant relationship with Alzheimer's disease, one would expect to see this disease cropping up in all those persons who have gastric disorders and are forced to take various antacid preparations. Since this is not the case, I believe that the relationship between aluminum ingestion and Alzheimer's disease is not substantiated.

What about alcohol consumption? Is there any link between use of alcohol and the onset of Alzheimer's? Indirect evidence exists about the connection between brain injury and Alzheimer's disease, and of course brain injury can in turn be caused by alcohol abuse. In addition, factors such as vitamin deficiencies and seizures stemming from alcoholism tend to confound the role of alcohol abuse in producing various syndromes that entail memory loss. There is evidence, however, that brain poisoning by alcohol can in itself reduce memory power. Alcohol-related dementia associated with atrophy of the brain and major loss of intellectual power, including vital memory, can also occur, though usually at a much younger age than Alzheimer's disease.

But although new discoveries have yielded tantalizing clues, I repeat that we don't yet know the exact cause of Alzheimer's disease and therefore have no sure method of prevention. This situation may well change in the next five years, but for now we can only hope that funding of basic research continues until a breakthrough comes.

Reducing Our Risk of Memory Loss

Brain Injury   We don't know enough yet to make specific recommendations for preventing Alzheimer's disease, but the risk factors for some other serious threats are only too well known.

Of utmost importance is the prevention of serious brain injury. Over half a million people in the United States suffer brain injuries related to automobile accidents each year; one hundred thousand of these injuries are serious. One of the most effective preventive measures is to have air bags fitted into every vehicle on the streets and highways of this country. Air bags, along with the use of three-point seat belt restraints, would markedly diminish the incidence of brain injuries. In addition, requiring appropriate helmets to be worn by players in all contact sports as well as by anyone riding a two- or three-wheel vehicle would be of great help.

And to take a public health approach to a grievous social problem, we should make every effort to lower the incidence of a mounting source of brain injury: gunshot wounds to the head. The streets of many American cities have become like war zones, with random shootings devastating the lives of not only those dealing in illegal drugs but also innocent bystanders. In the armed services, metal helmets are worn to reduce the velocity of bullets and shrapnel; instead of a high-velocity missile injury of the brain, a low-velocity missile wound results if the fragment penetrates the metal helmet, with consequent reduction in brain injury. What should we do in our urban areas? Issue infantry helmets to the residents — men, women, and children of the inner city? Perhaps a more effective proposal would be to license persons who have guns of any sort inside the limits of our major urban areas, with severe penalties for anyone caught with an unlicensed gun.

Brain Poisoning What role does brain poisoning play in premature loss of intellectual and memory functions? A very large one, in my view, among the more than six million alcoholics in this country as well as the millions who abuse cocaine, marijuana, Angel Dust, amphetamines, barbiturates, and other street drugs. Brain function is obviously impaired during the acute period of brain poisoning by alcohol or any of the street drugs, which cause a breakdown of the blood-brain barrier. This impairment can be as severe as that produced by a brain tumor, brain injury, or brain infection; the only difference is that brain function will return once the level of poisoning has abated. The chronic use of these brain poisons, however, is associated with the early onset of memory loss and deterioration of other intellectual powers. As I see it, the less these poisons are used, the better.

You should also try to minimize the use of various brain toxins that are medically prescribed, particularly the sedative hypnotics such as Ativan, Valium, Xanax, and Halcion as well as the barbiturates, the bromides, and the major psychiatric drugs such as Stelazine, haloperidol, Thorazine, and lithium. In addition, drugs used in general medicine — digitalis, pain relievers, drugs used to control hypertension and diabetes, cimetidine, beta blockers (such as Inderal), Reserpine, Symmetrel, and drugs like Elavil that have anticholinergic actions (that is, are antagonistic to the neurotransmitter acetylcholine) — are potentially toxic to brain and memory function.

Obviously, you should not abandon medications prescribed by your doctor, even psychiatric medications, if they're clinically indicated. If you are losing memory or are having periods of confusion, however, you should go to your doctor and ask that the dosage be adjusted so you still get the therapeutic effect without the toxic or adverse reactions some of these drugs produce. Also, at times it's possible for your physician to substitute one drug for another to achieve the same therapeutic effect without the toxic side effect on the brain. Moreover, if you're taking a number of drugs for various medical problems, be sure your doctor knows about all the medications you're on, because sometimes combinations of drugs are more toxic to the brain than a single drug alone. Combinations of Mellaril and lithium or haloperidol and methyldopa, for example, are especially likely to produce loss of memory, confusion, and intellectual deterioration. Among the drugs reviewed should be eye drops for glaucoma and skin patches to prevent seasickness.

It is also important to avoid chemicals and pollutants in auto emissions and industrial waste products. Carbon dioxide, carbon monoxide, organic solvents, mercury, lead, and arsenic are simply a few of the many poisons that can contaminate our air, food chain, and water supply and adversely affect brain function and memory.

Diet and Memory Loss

Another frequently asked question about prevention is, "What about diet? Is what I eat important in keeping me mentally alert?" The answer is an unequivocal yes. Diet is crucial at all stages of the life cycle, especially during the prenatal period and in infancy, when the developing brain is extremely sensitive to nutritional deficiencies. Serial studies have shown that a lack of essential nutrients can affect certain neurotransmitter systems in the brain at the earliest stages of life, and the damage is never really fully corrected even when an adequate diet is initiated.

TABLE 2 **Recommended Daily Minimum and Optimal Allowances of Vitamins and Minerals (For Adults and Children Ten Years Old and Older)[a]**

	Minimum	*Optimal*
Vitamins		
Vitamin A	5000 IU[b]	10,000 IU
Vitamin D	400 IU	400 IU
Vitamin E	30 IU	400 IU
Vitamin C	60.0 mg	1000.0 mg
Vitamin B$_1$ (thiamine)	1.5 mg	20.0 mg
Vitamin B$_2$ (riboflavin)	1.7 mg	10.0 mg

269

Table 2 continued

	Minimum	Optimal
Vitamin B$_3$ (niacin)	20.0 mg	250.0 mg
Vitamin B$_5$ (pantothenic acid)	10.0 mg	20.0 mg
Vitamin B$_6$ (pyridoxine)	2.0 mg	20.0 mg
Vitamin B$_9$ (folic acid)	400.0 mcg	800.0 mcg
Vitamin B$_{12}$ (cobalamines)	6.0 mcg	400.0 mcg
Vitamin H[c] (biotin)	n/a	300.0 mcg
Choline[d]	n/a	1.0 g
Minerals		
Calcium[e]	1.0 g	1.6 g
Phosphorus[e]	1.0 g	1.6 g
Iodine	150.0 mcg	150.0 mcg
Iron	18.0 mg	20.0 mg
Magnesium	400.0 mg	400.0 mg
Copper	2.0 mg	3.0 mg
Zinc	15.0 mg	25.0 mg
Other		
Spring water	n/a	1.5–2.0 liters (45–60 oz.)

[a]For persons who do not have allergies to specific foods containing these vitamins and for those who don't have diabetes or liver, thyroid, or kidney disease. Vitamin or nutritional supplements may be necessary for people who have allergies or intolerances to foods like milk, cheese, nuts, or fish. Nonallergenic food supplements are available and are strongly recommended to overcome the potential nutritional deficiencies that would otherwise occur in persons intolerant to basic foods.

[b]IU stands for international units, an international standard for measuring quantities of substances such as vitamins.

[c]Various amounts of this vitamin are normally produced in the intestine.

[d]Many nutritionists do not consider choline to be a vitamin because some amount of it is produced in the body, but I consider it so important that you may need to supplement it.

[e]You may substitute 3.2 grams per day of calcium phosphate.

Many nutritionists will tell you that it's not necessary to take dietary supplements if your intake of cereals and grains, vegetables and fruits, milk products, and meat and fish is adequate. The unfortunate thing is that our lifestyles may preclude getting an adequate diet. Fast foods and processed foods may not contain the nourishment you need for your brain. Furthermore, as we get older we tend to be more sedentary and use fewer calories, so we eat less food, and the essential vitamins and nutrients may therefore be lacking in sufficient quantity. In addition, some people lose teeth as they grow older, and as a result they can't chew food properly and derive the full nutritional benefit from what they do eat.

I don't believe in megadoses of vitamins, but I also think that the optimal level of vitamins is greater than the classical nutritionists state. Therefore, I recommend the daily vitamin supplements listed in Table 2. These substances form the basis of adequate supplemental nutrition for the brain. In addition, I myself like to take a supplement of purified choline (phosphatidyl choline, or lecithin). I realize that some choline is manufactured in the body, and that the statistical evidence that this substance enhances memory is equivocal. However, I believe it helps. Tom Sabin introduced me to choline as a dietary supplement. After I started taking it, I felt as though my memory for names, and particularly the individual histories of patients, improved. This may be a placebo effect, and it may not reflect any direct change in the memory process but rather an improvement in my ability to concentrate and focus my attention so that new memories or engrams are encoded more efficiently.

There is some statistical evidence that choline does have an effect on memory in normal people. For example, a 1979 scientifically controlled study done at the National Institutes of Health showed that a dietary addition of 10 grams of choline a day did have an obvious effect on some components of memory. Two different tests were used to study the effects on learning and memory in normal volunteers whose average age was twenty-four. The first was an uncategorized serial learning test, and the second was a selective reminding test. In the first test, the subjects took fewer trials to learn a list of ten unrelated words after taking choline, and under the effects of choline the poorer performers showed greater improvement than the good performers.

In the first trial of the selective reminding test, a twelve-word list of common English words was read, half of which were high-imagery words, such as chair, and half of which were low-imagery words, such as lie. On successive trials the only words read were those not correctly recalled on the previous trial. Learning and recall were repeated until all the subjects said all twelve words perfectly on two successive trials, or until the trials had been done twelve times. The results showed that choline improved the storage and recall only of low-imagery words. Words recalled correctly on one trial were more likely to be recalled correctly on the next trial if they followed the administration of choline rather than a placebo.

Although the beneficial effect of choline on the memory of young people was consistent in this study, tests of the effect of choline in enhancing the memory of older people have been variable in their results. However, in 1996 a research group at Massachusetts Institute of Technology conducted an investigation into the effects of choline in older volunteers, especially with respect to the possible beneficial properties of a drug called citicoline.

The MIT researchers conducted several double-blind placebo-controlled studies of the effect that citicoline had on verbal memory. After data analysis, a subgroup was identified whose members had relatively inefficient memories. The subjects were recruited for a second study that used a crossover design. They took either a placebo or citicoline, 1000 mg a day, for three months in the initial study. In the crossover study, the subjects took both a placebo and citicoline, 2000 mg per day, each for two months. (The subjects were forty-seven female and forty-eight male volunteers, fifty to eighty-five years of age, who were screened for dementia, memory problems, and other neurological problems.) Of the subjects with relatively inefficient memories, thirty-two participated in the crossover study.

Verbal memory was tested at each study visit using a logical memory passage. Plasma choline concentrations and memory scores were analyzed using repeated measures of analysis of variance and covariance, followed by planned comparisons when appropriate.

In the initial study, citicoline therapy improved delayed recall on logical memory only for the subjects with relatively inefficient memories. In the crossover study, the higher dosage of citicoline was clearly associated with improved immediate and delayed logical memory.

There are several things to remember about these choline studies. First, choline is not a magic drug that will miraculously improve all aspects of your memory. The fact that the successful choline experiments have had a very selective effect on certain aspects of memory is somewhat reassuring, in that the results of the studies are genuine. Memory is a very complex process, however, involving a number of different brain functions. It is not logical to suppose that all of the brain processes related to memory would respond to choline. Second, the variability of the responses in volunteers and patients is in line with the kinds of effects that we get with other drugs, agents, or chemicals that affect the brain.

Returning to vitamins, in formulating our vitamin preparation, we specifically wanted to avoid including excessive levels of vitamins because, for example, too much pyridoxine (vitamin B-6) causes a disorder of the sensory part of the nervous system, especially in the ganglia situated alongside the spinal cord. We also did not include excitatory amino acids, like glutamic acid, in this formula, since in normal circumstances a transport system in the blood-brain barrier moves excess glutamic acid away from brain cells. If the transport system fails because of a breakdown in the blood-brain barrier, too much glutamic acid will accumulate around brain cells, leading to a concentration of calcium ions and the death of brain cells.

I also recommend that you drink forty-five to sixty ounces of pure water a day, provided kidney and heart function are normal.* Of course, fruit juices or skimmed milk (for those who do not have lactose intolerance) can be substituted for water.

What about people with a family history of early heart disease or stroke? Such persons should reduce the total amount of fat in their diets, relying chiefly on fish, chicken, and turkey (without the skin) and vegetables, such as beans, to supply protein. Deep-sea fish, such as salmon and tuna, are particularly good choices because of the essential fatty acids they contain. Most kinds of high-fat meat should be avoided. Eggs — hard- or soft-boiled — have good nutritional value, even though they do contain cholesterol; one or two can be eaten once or twice a week. Avoid butter, margarine made with hydrogenated oil, peanut butter made with hydrogenated oil, ice cream, cream, whole milk, desserts made with lard or vegetable shortening, and foods fried in lard or shortening. Of course, the diet should contain substantial amounts of fruit and vegetables.

There is now clear evidence that omega-3 fatty acid is essential for normal eye and brain development in the fetus. This is also true for pre-term infants. Mother's milk provides an ideal source of essential fatty acids to help premature infants avoid abnormal brain and retinal development. There is also a ques-

---

*I drink bottled water because tap water in many locations contains an excessive amount of chlorine, which may injure the bladder lining.

tion as to whether there should be fatty acid supplementation of the diets of pregnant women to avoid fetal abnormalities of the brain and heart. Eating oily fish in pregnancy has been found to have a slight but definite beneficial effect on the birth weight and length of gestation of newborns. The addition of oily fish to the diet, for example, kippers, herring, mackerel, salmon, sardines, or tuna, twice or three times a week, can be encouraged as part of a healthy balanced diet in pregnancy, and for the whole family.

Even though omega-3 fatty acids are important for normal brain development, however, there is no evidence that the fatty acids and the fish that contain them have any part in reducing strokes. A study was done in the department of neurology at Northwestern University medical school on a group of over 2,000 men aged forty to fifty-five to test this point. Those men who consumed the most fish did *not*, in fact, have a reduction in their incidence of stroke.

It has been known for some time that a diet high in fat, and especially a diet high in saturated fat, is associated with an increased incidence of coronary heart disease. A recent study done at the Harvard University school of public health, however, showed that replacing saturated fat with monounsaturated and polyunsaturated fats is more effective in preventing coronary heart disease in women than reducing overall fat intake.

There is a great deal of clinical evidence that there is an association between heart attacks and stroke. Often, one follows the other. Thus, as mentioned before, a recent report from the Harvard medical school, relying upon the population-based study called the Framingham heart study, was most surprising and inexplicable. The study found that higher intakes of fat, saturated fat, and monosaturated fat were associated with reduced risk of nonhemorrhagic stroke in men. Also, a California study found that higher serum levels of the essential fatty acid alpha linolenic acid were independently associated with a lower risk of stroke in middle-aged men at high risk for cardiovascular disease.

My conclusions from all of the currently available evidence is that an increased intake of monounsaturated fatty acids, such as canola oil, olive oil, and even a modest amount of peanut oil, is helpful in avoiding both cardiovascular disease and stroke. I also believe that when this dietary controversy is resolved, oily fish in the diet will be found to be helpful in avoiding cardiovascular disease and promoting healthy brain function.

Because hypertension is often associated with early heart disease and stroke, a diet low in sodium should be initiated — which means not merely not adding table salt but also avoiding many canned foods and soups, which are loaded with sodium. Moreover, control the total number of calories taken in if weight is a problem. Olive oil and vinegar dressings with condiments such as garlic and onions added are preferable to commercial high-calorie salad dressings, and soybean desserts, such as low-fat Tofutti, taste like ice cream but have almost no fat and reduced calories. Also, although this item isn't strictly related to diet, people with heart disease or stroke in their families should avoid the use of tobacco.

Contrary to the usual practice of Americans, it is advisable that you eat your largest meal in the morning, including fish, chicken, or turkey; you can then snack during the day on low-fat foods like vegetables and fruits and have a very small amount to eat at night just before going to bed, when the calories taken in will not be used up immediately.

Another sure way to avoid weight gain is to buy a doctor's scale. Unlike inaccurate spring scales, shifting weight from one foot to another on a balance beam scale will not reduce your weight by five to eight pounds. If you are gaining weight or not losing it as you'd like, it means one thing: you have to cut down on your food intake. Losing extra pounds can be more difficult for some people than for others if they have a genetic predisposition to being overweight. Even so, the body is fundamentally a heat machine. To maintain constant weight, calories in must equal calories out. If we take in more calories than we use up, we will store the excess as fat in our bodies. Generally speaking, people who weigh less are less prone to heart attacks and strokes than those who are overweight.

Exercise and Health

Will exercise help us avoid the kind of strokes associated with hardening of the arteries or arteriosclerotic disease? Yes, I believe it will, but that doesn't mean you have to be able to run a six-minute mile, or swim three hundred yards every morning, or go into a weight room for a forty-five-minute daily workout. As we get older our joints are more susceptible to injury from vigorous exercise, so I suggest any of the following programs to be done on a daily basis:

- walking or bicycling for forty-five minutes a day (walking to be done at three to four miles an hour)
- swimming for twenty to thirty minutes a day
- gentle jogging for twelve to fifteen minutes a day
- gentle resistance exercises and calisthenics for ten minutes a day

Keeping the body musculature toned up with calisthenic exercises is important. It's especially helpful to do sit-ups with the knees bent so that the abdominal muscles remain firm and strong and no undue strain is put on the back muscles. If one then has an occasional accidental fall, the body posture can be maintained by strong abdominal muscles aiding the back muscles in protecting against serious back and head injury.

Less demanding aerobic exercises like walking have to be done for a longer period of time than, say, running to get the same effect. But unlike some experts, who are satisfied with seeing people exercise three times a week, I believe in exercising daily — but I run only a mile and a half, not five miles.

What effect does exercise itself have on memory function? A few studies have been done. French physiologists investigated the influence of physical exercise on simple reaction time. They tested two groups of ten subjects each. One group consisted of trained middle-distance runners, and the other group was made up of students who had no regular physical training.

The subjects performed a simple reaction time test while pedaling on an exercise bicycle at relative powers corresponding to 20, 40, 60, and 80 percent of their own maximal aerobic power, and immediately after exercise. During exercise, the results showed a decrease in intellectual and memory performance for both groups, but no significant effect was found after exercise. (A significant positive effect of physical fitness on simple reaction time was noted during exercise.)

Researchers in the Netherlands studied a population of different ages unselected for aerobic fitness. The physical fitness of the subjects with respect to age was correlated with the performance on intelligence and memory tests. Those participants who engaged in aerobic sports felt healthier than participants who did not, and they did better on certain intellectual tests. (An additional study by this group found age effects on several measures of intellectual speed and fluency but not on memory performance.)

Finally, another study to determine the effects of exercise on learning and memory was carried out at the University of Wales. Participants in these studies learned lists of words in two physiological states: at rest and while exercising on a bicycle. Word lists learned during the aerobic exercise were recalled best during aerobic exercise. Recall levels for words both learned and recalled during exercise were equal to those levels for words both learned and recalled at rest. These findings appear to rule out the possibility that exercise interferes with original learning.

Brain Exercises

Are there any specific brain exercises that can be done to help you improve or retain memory? Yes, and they are of several kinds. The first are preventive to make sure that as much brain function is retained after brain injuries or strokes as possible, and to aid in the rehabilitation process. Examples of these exercises are learning to write, or at least print, with the nondominant hand (usually the left); learning to get visual cues from the left visual field; and shaving or brushing one's teeth with the nondominant hand. Of course, such learning is much more effective if it's done before the age of five. But even in old age it has some protective effect if it is done before a stroke or injury.

Practicing all aspects of intellectual function and improving them as much as possible, although they aren't absolute preventives as far as Alzheimer's disease is concerned, certainly help to slow down the brain's aging process in the normal individual. Math skills should be practiced, including balancing your checkbook without a calculator. Drawing with either hand, reading, and particularly reading aloud should also be a part of your mental practice.

More specific exercises to hone memory skills should focus on attention, concentration, and avoiding distraction. (Ideally, such skills should be practiced from kindergarten on, but it's never too late to begin. A complete program of these exercises can be found in my previous book, *Brain Power*.) In exercises to improve attention, an individual estimates the amount of time that has gone by and is checked by an observer with a stopwatch, concentrating enough to estimate intervals of ten seconds, twenty seconds, sixty seconds.

In another set of exercises, an examiner shows the subject various letters of the alphabet and associates each with a number. The subject is given time to memorize the letters and their corresponding numbers, which represent increments of time. The examiner then holds up a letter and instructs the subject to stop a watch when the elapsed time equals the numerical value of the letter.

A number of memory exercises, though they have not been effective in rehabilitating brain-injured people, do help expand the memory functions of normal individuals. These exercises enhance the ability to retain certain memories, and anyone can potentially profit from their use. Based on the association method of memory (sometimes called mnemonics), they involve correlating items to be remembered with other known information. Using these techniques, however, is like learning French or algebra: it requires time and concentration. The several varieties of mnemonics do work, sometimes in a spectacular fashion, but you must keep practicing them. Once you discover a memory technique that works for you, incorporate it into a short daily exercise routine.

Besides physical and mental exercises, your routine should include brain relaxation exercises. Relaxation doesn't mean allowing yourself to crumple into a heap and allow whatever unwarranted or unwanted thoughts that are on the scene to parade through your mind. It means excluding everything that's going on in your environment, usually by sitting in a darkened room in a semireclining position with your eyes closed and a minimum of noise around you, and practicing a concentration technique to focus your attention.

Many different methods of relaxation are available, including autohypnosis, which is part of the conditioned reflex program defined by psychologist Andrew Salter; the "relaxation response" to induce lower blood pressure, written about by Herbert Benson; the system of Transcendental Meditation; and a number of other similar techniques.

One method I have advocated for achieving brain relaxation takes advantage of the physiological fact that certain portions of the anatomy, particularly the lips, tongue, index fingers, and great toes, are better represented on the surface of the brain (the cortex) than are other anatomical structures. To try this technique, eliminate all distractions and sit quietly with your eyes closed in the relaxation position. Focus your attention on relaxing the tip of your right thumb and work backward to the first joint, then the second. Concentrate on the anatomical structure of your thumb. After thirty to sixty seconds have passed, repeat the exercise, this time focusing on the middle and little fingers of your right hand. When you're finished with your right hand you can begin on your left; then on the right part of your tongue, the tip of the tongue, and the left part of the tongue; then on the muscles around your lips. Proceed to the eyelids on the right, first the upper, then the lower, and then transfer to the left side. If you're not completely relaxed at this time, go to the toes on your feet, beginning with the great toe on your right side.

Don't start these relaxation exercises when you're tense or upset; doing so will cause you to form bad conditioned reflexes, and the relaxation will not work. Rather, practice them first when you are relaxed so you can develop strong conditioned reflexes, which can eventually be applied in stressful situations. In my opinion relaxation exercises should be interspersed with memory exercises to achieve the best results. I also suggest that they be done in conjunction with physical exercises and mental exercises involving other parts of the brain, such as drawing, reading, and calculating.

Finally, to maintain brain fitness it is important to focus your attention on other people and other things. In any case, do not focus your attention on yourself. The more you think of yourself — your pleasures, what's in it for you — the more apt you are to become bored, fatigued, and ultimately depressed, with the kind of depression accompanied by hypochondriasis, easy distractibility, and loss of memory. This is the lesson taught by Mother Teresa, Dr. Albert Schweitzer, and St. Francis of Assisi. Never give up your interest in other people and other things. Always accept outside challenges as long as they are matched by your own talents and enthusiasm.

Since this book was first published in 1992, new information has become available about the effects of certain chemicals and biologicals on preserving and enhancing memory function. There is now considerable evidence from basic neuroscience that estrogen influences aspects of brain chemistry and brain morphology known to be important for memory functions. For example, studies of menopausal women have demonstrated that taking additional estrogen enhanced short- and long-term memory and the capacity for learning new associations, while having little effect on visual memory.

There are, in fact, a number of case reports of women sixty-five years of age performing better on memory tests after being medicated with estrogen than did matched controls who were estrogen-nonusers. Overall, there are a number of studies suggesting that medicating post-menopausal women with estrogen helps to maintain verbal memory and enhances the capacity for new learning.

Estrogen replacement therapy has also been proposed as a protective factor against developing Alzheimer's disease. Some scientists hypothesize that estrogen effects may be mediated by estrogen receptors in the basal forebrain and hippocampus, effects on cholinergic neurotransmission, modulation of levels of neurotropic growth factors, and maintenance of synaptic density.

A somewhat controversial study was carried out in 1997 at Case Western Reserve University's Alzheimer's center in Cleveland to determine the effects of estrogen replacement therapy and smoking history, and an assessment of the interaction of estrogen replacement therapy with cigarette smoking as a protective factor against Alzheimer's disease. The study population consisted of 88 women with Alzheimer's disease and 176 matched healthy women as controls. Data were obtained for the teenage years and each twenty-year period of adulthood starting from the twenties and thirties to the present by use of self-administered questionnaires for the controls. Alzheimer's disease patients' data were obtained from caregivers with the same questionnaire, assaying life history until five years before the onset of Alzheimer's disease.

Ironically, considering all the negative effects of smoking, the study showed the possibility of a synergistic protective effect of estrogen replacement therapy and smoking cigarettes against the development of Alzheimer's disease. It is obvious to those who have smoked cigarettes that nicotine has a substantial effect on brain function. It is not surprising then that pronounced nicotinic receptors dysfunction, and impaired semantic memory, occur early in the course of Alzheimer's disease. Clinical research has indicated that nicotine has the ability to enhance alertness, arousal, and other mental functions in normal people. It has been postulated that this effect is a function of its ability to stimulate central nervous system nicotinic cholinergic receptors.

In a study carried out at Southern Illinois University school of medicine on patients with early Alzheimer's disease and on elderly normal people, the participants underwent PET scanning during a verbal fluency challenge procedure using nicotine. The results of this double-blind study showed that with the administration of nicotine there was an increase in regional cerebral glucose metabolism in the Alzheimer patients but not in the controls. Verbal fluency scores increased by an average of 17 percent in the Alzheimer patients. (This is a measure of semantic memory.) The study produced objective data on the effect of nicotine administration on the function of the brain. As such, it increases the reliability of psychometric tests that show improvement in semantic memory.

There are a number of food additives that are said to improve memory. These include a vitamin called substance P, the effects of which were predicted by animal experiments. Substance P does appear to contain certain chemical constituents similar to those found in red wine, but there's not much hard evidence for its being useful in improving human memory.

Another chemical substance that may have a beneficial effect on memory is called actovegin. It is a protein-free metabolically active hemo (blood) derivative that improves oxygen and glucose utilization. People who received this agent in one study had an improvement in the electrical potentials of their brain.

A drug called Taxol is now being investigated because of its potential for protecting neurons in the brain against beta-amyloid toxicity. Theoretically, this compound could preserve memory by interrupting one of the destructive chemical sequences in the brain produced by Alzheimer's disease.

Looking at the prevention of Alzheimer's disease as a method of preserving memory, it is useful to note that a number of longitudinal studies are being carried out in terms of reducing the risk of developing Alzheimer's disease. Both steroids and nonsteroidal anti-inflammatory drugs are being tested. We have already mentioned the nonsteroidal anti-inflammatory drugs. It is worthwhile noting that in addition to these agents steroids such as dexamethasone are also being tested in this regard.

The efficacy of ginko biloba has been tested in patients suffering from mild to moderate Alzheimer's disease, and in patients who have multi-infarct dementia. At the University of Berlin a randomized double-blind placebo-controlled multi-center study was done. After a four-week acclimatization, 216 patients were included in the randomized twenty-four-week treatment period. They received either a daily oral dose of 240 mg of ginko biloba, or a placebo. Three primary variables were chosen as test vehicles: the clinical global impressions for psycho-pathological assessment, tests to assess the patient's attention and memory, and a test to measure the activities of daily living.

The results of these tests from the 156 patients who completed the study showed beneficial effects of the ginko biloba administration in people with the dementia of Alzheimer's disease, as well as in people with multi-infarct dementia. These results were confirmed in another study of ginko biloba by the University Hospital department of psychiatry in Frankfurt, Germany. Ginko biloba was also found to have a beneficial effect by neurologists in Lucknow, India, in patients with acute ischemic stroke.

Pregnenolone sulfate is another agent that has demonstrated promising results in experimental animals, as far as memory is concerned. It is postulated from animal studies that pregnenolone sulfate will have a more potent effect on memory than dehydroepiandrosterone sulfate or corticosterone. (A more complete explanation of these effects was covered in an earlier section on hormones.)

Vital Memory Points to Remember

1. Using appropriate brain exercises to keep your brain challenged and active will help maintain brain health.
2. The best way to reduce the risk of brain injury and memory loss is through having air bags installed and using three-point safety belts in automobiles.
3. Avoiding brain poisons of all kinds will greatly reduce your chance of suffering memory loss.
4. Dietary supplements, particularly of certain B vitamins, can help people who are concerned about memory loss from malnutrition.

22

Predictions: Preventing and Reversing Memory Loss

Alzheimer's Disease

WE WILL HAVE effective treatments for some forms of Alzheimer's disease in the next twenty years.* I believe that many of the necessary technical tools will be available in ten years, but population testing and government regulations may extend the time required to make these treatments available to all patients.

Alzheimer's is the most frequent irreversible cause of memory loss in the elderly, and its effective treatment will depend on early and accurate diagnosis, which, I predict, will take place in three years.

Beta amyloid protein, a complex of forty-two amino acids, is associated with brain cell death in Alzheimer's disease. This protein is present beneath the skin in Alzheimer's patients, and an abnormal amyloid protein, A-68, is found in patients' spinal fluid. I believe that either a spinal fluid examination or a skin biopsy will be the method used to confirm the diagnosis of Alzheimer's. Perhaps a monoclonal antibody will be used as a detector.

*The predictions in this chapter are based on the assumption that sufficient financial support will be available to carry out the necessary research.

The memory loss in Alzheimer's disease is correlated with a reduction in levels of the neurotransmitter acetylcholine in areas of the brain where new memories are formed. New drugs are now being introduced to increase the amount of acetylcholine in the brain.

I predict that we will develop chemicals that will promote the survival and growth of nerve cells. One of these may be a genetically engineered nerve cell growth factor.* Furthermore, I predict that within ten years we will be able to transplant fetal brain cells or stem cells into the brains of Alzheimer's patients to replace their dead or dying cells. I believe that we will be able to harvest and grow such cells in cell cultures located in cell banks across the country. Through advances in genetic engineering, these cells will be transplanted into the host without the need for immunosuppressant drugs to inactivate the body's immune system so the cells will not be rejected.

New drugs will be developed to keep brain cells from being destroyed. Drugs already in use prevent brain cell death from excess calcium ions, but I predict that within the next five years drugs or a vaccine that will inhibit the enzyme activity essential for the buildup of beta amyloid, the compound that may be responsible for nerve cell death in Alzheimer's, will be available.

Researchers will find more than one gene connected to Alzheimer's disease, and on the basis of genetic classification alone we will find that what we now know as Alzheimer's disease actually comprises at least three different diseases, each with a different cause and treatment.

Finally, the recent discovery of living stem cells in the brain of adult human beings raises the possibility of finding some way of stimulating such cells so that they will repair or replace injured brain cells in patients with Alzheimer's disease or stroke. Since these primitive stem cells are multi-potential,

*A promising drug with these properties, called Neotrophin, is now being tested in patients with early Alzheimer's disease by a company called Neotherapeutics.

they would probably be able to repair or replace any brain cell, no matter how specialized it is. In fact, this discovery may well inaugurate a new era in the treatment of brain and spinal cord injury and disease.

Multi-Infarct Dementia (Small Strokes)

I predict that we will reduce the incidence and severity of multi-infarct dementia, the second leading cause of irreversible memory loss in the elderly, in the next eight years. We will develop noninvasive tests to determine who is at risk for the disease, and we will develop new antihypertensive medications that will carry a smaller risk of low blood pressure in the blood vessels of the brain than that posed by the agents now in use.

We will have emergency techniques to unplug occluded blood vessels in the brain while they are in the process of producing an acute stroke. Such a technique might be to immediately insert a catheter into the blocked blood vessels and squirt in a clot-dissolving liquid, or to insert a fiberoptic scope into the blood vessel and pulverize the clot with either a new kind of laser or focused ultrasound, neither of which will damage the blood vessel wall.

New medications will be developed to reverse the arteriosclerotic process that results in narrowing of blood vessels. I believe this will be a boon to many Americans, who won't have gone on low-fat diets, even though high-fat diets endanger their health.

Within the next twenty years, genetic engineering will enable doctors to change the genetic makeup of those of us whose genes make us susceptible to early heart attack and stroke. Without restricting our diets, we will be able to maintain clean, healthy arteries and live vigorously into advanced old age.

The Brain as an Electrochemical System

Within the next twenty years you're going to see many people walking around with electrodes strapped to their scalps. They will look as though they have tape players piping music into their ears, but it won't be music playing. Instead, electrodes will deliver electrical or electromagnetic currents to their heads. These tiny currents will increase the level of certain neurotransmitters in the spinal fluid, such as serotonin or dopamine, and will not only reverse depression but also correct associated memory problems.

These electrodes will reduce the amount of prescription tranquilizers and street drugs consumed by people. It should also entirely eliminate the need for drugs that have toxic effects on the brain. I do not advocate that people who aren't ill use transcranial electrical brain stimulation. But once people understand that their brains are electrochemical mechanisms that can be influenced by electrical current as well as by chemicals or drugs, it may be impossible to stop the widespread use of such devices to promote a feeling of relaxation.

Very weak transcranial electrical stimulation was first experimented with in the late fifties. Soviet doctors used it as an anesthetic, and in this country two psychiatrists reversed depression in severely depressed patients resistant to medication.

In 1965, Frank Ervin, Sol Aranow, and I applied very weak direct currents to the scalps of depressed patients. The currents had no effect in about a third of the patients, a transient beneficial effect in another third, and profound effects in reversing depression in the last third. These weak electrical currents produced changes in the brain's electromagnetic field, which in turn generated a current that stimulated the limbic portions of the brain. In patients who had a striking improvement in their depression, we found that the direction of flow of the direct current was important in producing the beneficial effect. Reversing the direction of flow reversed the effect on the patients' depression.

An inventor and electrical engineer, Mr. Sol Liss, observing some of the work going on in our laboratory, altered an electronic device he had invented for transcutaneous electrical stimulation of nerves to relieve pain. In effect, he invented a new kind of cranial-stimulating device which supplied current in tiny amounts.

The Future of Transcranial Electrical Brain Stimulation

Evidence is mounting that transcranial electrical brain stimulation can decrease drug dependence in abusers of some drugs, including heroin, cocaine, alcohol, and even prescription drugs. I predict that this technique will be widely used in the treatment of drug dependency in the next five years.

Since this kind of electrical stimulation seems to relieve depression (often present in drug and alcohol abusers) as one of its primary modes of action, the loss of memory associated with depression, produced by hyperdistractibility — the inability to concentrate or focus attention — should be relieved. Especially in persons over forty-five who have mild depression and complain of memory loss, transcranial stimulation may be of significant value. I predict that in the next five to ten years transcranial electrical brain stimulation will become an important treatment for depression and its associated memory loss.

Dr. Allan Chiles of Austin, Texas, who directs a rehabilitation hospital for the severely brain-injured, has recently reported that transcranial electrical stimulation has helped to reduce the memory loss of several patients with persistent post-traumatic amnesia. I predict that within the next ten years transcranial electrical stimulation will help rouse stuporous, brain-injured patients into consciousness.

Finally, I predict that new discoveries about the frequencies and intensities of electrical currents and electromagnetic fields will allow them to be focused on the head in such a way as to selectively stimulate both deep and superficial areas of the brain in the treatment of a number of psychiatric and neurobehavioral symptoms. I predict that transcranial electrical brain stimulation will become widely used by physicians in psychiatry and rehabilitation medicine.

A recent issue of the *Harvard University Gazette* featured the work of associate professor Pascual-Leone. The writer was impressed with this doctor's ability to make a depressed person feel good just by waving a wand over his or her head. He could also speed up the slow, stiff movements of a patient with Parkinson's disease, and the doctor's magnetic wand also helped schizophrenic and obsessive-compulsive patients control their behavior. It could even push blind people to learn Braille more quickly.

Dr. Leone, his colleagues at the National Institutes of Health, and neurologists in a number of university hospital settings have experimented with the effects of magnetic and electrical fields on the brain for more than a decade. Their research shows that magnetic fields from a hand-held magnetic wand generate electrical currents in a person's brain. Furthermore, such currents can help us determine how the brain works. Neurologists at the National Institutes of Health have used this tool to map the locations of brain areas that control language, memory, and attention. They also showed how these functions can be blocked or enhanced when electrical currents increase or decrease the activity of selected brain cells.

The electromagnetic wand generates a magnetic field when electric coils and capacitors are switched on and off rapidly. The magnetic field, in turn, induces secondary electric currents in the brain. It works much like a transformer. Dr. Leone and other neurologists around the country have used this technique to successfully treat patients with severe depression.

The kind of clinical experiment that I am about to describe is important in the treatment of memory disorders because depression is one of the most frequent causes of memory impairment. Depression produces hyperdistractibility, inability to concentrate, and an inability to lay down new memories. It also interferes with the storage of memory and its later retrieval.

In one set of experiments, stimulating the left frontal brain improved the moods of eleven out of seventeen badly depressed patients. According to Dr. Leone, these patients had not been helped by drugs or even electro-shock treatment. If the stimulation was carried out for five to ten days, the beneficial mood improvement could be extended up to several months.

The advantage of the electromagnetic brain stimulation over other forms of brain stimulation is the precision with which this stimulation can be carried out. The desired areas of the brain to be stimulated can be activated without stimulating surrounding areas of the brain. In addition, substantial amounts of current can be applied to the head without producing pain.

There is much work that needs to be done before electromagnetic stimulation of the brain will become a standard therapy. However, we can definitely see light at the end of the tunnel. This therapy holds much promise, and more importantly, appears to pose little risk to the patient.

Conclusions and Summary

1. Loss of vital memory isn't part of normal aging.
2. True loss of vital memory means that you have a physical problem and need medical assessment.
3. A memory problem can best be defined by memory testing and a neurological examination.
4. Early diagnosis and prompt treatment can completely re-

verse many memory problems while making others less severe and more manageable.

5. There are methods to help you avoid memory problems and make your memory more efficient.
6. It is hoped that in a few years even the most severe memory problems will be treatable and, in another decade, preventable.

Bibliography

Scholarly Books and Articles

Adams, R. D., Victor, M. *Principles of Neurology.* 3rd ed. New York: McGraw-Hill, 1985.

Alvarez-Buylla, A., Kirn, J., and Nottebohm, F. "Birth of Projection Neurons in Adult Avian Brain May Be Related to Perceptual or Motor Learning." *Science* 249:1444–46, 1990.

Barnes, H. N., Aronson, M. D., and Delbanco, T. L., eds. *Alcoholism: A Guide for the Primary Care Physician.* New York: Springer-Verlag, 1987.

Beaton, G. H., and Bengoa, J. M., eds. *Nutrition in Preventive Medicine.* Geneva: World Health Organization, 1976.

Beatty, W. W. "Opiate Antagonists, Morphine and Spatial Memory in Rats." *Pharmacology, Biochemistry and Behavior* 19:397–401, 1983.

Blaney, P. H. "Affect and Memory: A Review." *Psychological Bulletin* 99:229–46, 1986.

Block, R. I., Wittenborn, J. R. "Marijuana Effects on the Speed of Memory Retrieval in the Letter-matching Task." *International Journal of the Addictions* 21:281–85, 1986.

——. "Marijuana Effects on Semantic Memory." *Psychological Reports* 55:503–512, 1984.

Bolla, K., et al. "Memory Complaints in Older Adults." *Archives of Neurology* 48:61–64, 1991.

Butters, N., Cermak, L. *Alcoholic Korsakoff's Syndrome.* New York: Academic Press, 1980.

Church, A. C., et al. "Long-Term Suppression of the Cerebral Spread of a Memory: Effects of Idazoxan and Clonidine." *Pharmacology, Biochemistry and Behavior* 32:749–56, 1989.

Croog, S., et al. "The Effects of Antihypertensive Therapy on the Quality of Life." *New England Journal of Medicine* 314:1657–64, 1986.

Davidoff, D. A., Kessler, H. R., Laibstain, D. F., Mark, V. H. "Neurobehavioral Sequelae of Minor Head Injury: A Consideration of Post-Concussive Syndrome Versus Past Traumatic Stress Disorder." *Cognitive Rehabilitation* (March/April):8–13, 1988.

Ellis, H. C. "On the Importance of Mood Intensity and Encoding Demands in Memory: Commentary on Hasher, Rose, Zacks, Sanft, and Doren." *Journal of Experimental Psychology* 114:392–95, 1985.

Ervin, F. R., Aranow, S., Mark, V. H. "Low Level DC Polarization in Man: Clinical Behavioral and Electrophysiologic Observations." *Abstracts of the Conference on Effects of Diffuse Electrical Currents on Physiological Mechanisms with Application to Electroanesthesia and Electrosleep* 4:23, 1966.

Fitten, L., et al. "Treatment of Alzheimer's Disease with Short- and Long-Term Oral THA and Lecithin." *American Journal of Psychiatry* 147:239–42, 1990.

Fossen, A., et al. "Effects of Hypnotics on Memory." *Pharmacology* 27, supp. 2:116–26, 1983.

Fulginiti, S., Cancela, L. "Effect of Naloxone and Amphetamine on Acquisition and Memory Consolidation of Active Avoidance Responses in Rats." *Psychopharmacology* 79:45–48, 1983.

Gawin, F. H., Ellingwood, E. H. "Cocaine and Other Stimulants." *New England Journal of Medicine* 318:1173–82, 1988.

Greenwood, C. "The Role of Diet in Modulating Brain Metabolism and Behavior." *Contemporary Nutrition* 14, no. 7, 1989.

Griffith, H. W. *Complete Guide to Vitamins, Minerals, and Supplements.* Tucson: Fisher, 1988.

Hall, S., Bornstein, R. "The Relationship Between Intelligence and Memory Following Minor or Mild Closed Head Injury." *Journal of Neurosurgery* 75:378–81, 1991.

Harrell, R. F. "Mental Response to Added Thiamine." *Journal of Nutrition* 31:283–98, 1946.

Hartley, L. R., et al. "The Effect of Beta Adrenergic Blocking Drugs on Speakers' Performance and Memory." *British Journal of Psychiatry* 142:512–17, 1983.

Hilton, H. *The Executive Memory Guide.* New York: Simon and Schuster, 1986.

Horn, J. L. "Psychometric Studies of Aging and Intelligence." In *Aging: Genesis and Treatment of Psychological Disorders in the Elderly*, edited by Gersons and Rankin, 19–43. New York: Raven Press, 1975.

Izquierdo, I., Graudenz, M. "Memory Facilitation by Naloxone Is Due to Release of Dopaminergic and Beta-Adrenergic Systems from Tonic Inhibition." *Psychopharmacology* 67:265–68, 1980.

Katzman, R., Terry, R. D., eds. *The Neurology of Aging.* Philadelphia: Davis, 1984.

Kirk, A., Kertesz, A. "On Drawing Impairment in Alzheimer's Disease." *Archives of Neurology* 48:73–77, 1991.

Kirk, R. C., White, K., McNaughton, N. "Low Dose Scopolamine Affects Discriminability but Not Rate of Forgetting in Delayed Conditional Discrimination." *Psychopharmacology* 96:541–46, 1988.

Lee, J. C. "The Effects of Alcohol Injections on the Blood-Brain Barrier." *Quarterly Journal of Studies on Alcohol* 23:4–16, 1962.

Loke, Wing H. "Effects of Caffeine on Mood and Memory." *Physiology and Behavior* 44:367–72, 1988.

Madrazo, L. V., et al. "Transplantation of Fetal Substantia Nigra and Adrenal Medulla to the Caudate Nucleus in Two Patients with Parkinson's Disease." *New England Journal of Medicine* 318:51, 1988.

Mark, V. H., et al. "The Destruction of Both Anterior Thalamic Nuclei in a Patient with Intractable Agitated Depression." *Journal of Nervous and Mental Disease* 150:266–72, 1970.

Bibliography

Mark, V. H., Ervin, F. R. *Violence and the Brain.* New York: Harper and Row, 1970.

Mark, V. H., Ervin, F., Sweet, W. "Deep Temporal Lobe Stimulation in Man." In *The Neurobiology of the Amygdala,* edited by Basil E. Eleftheriou, 485–507. New York: Plenum, 1971.

Mark, V. H., with J. P. Mark. *Brain Power.* Boston: Houghton Mifflin, 1989.

McGlone, J., et al. "Screening for Early Dementia Using Memory Complaints from Patients and Relatives." *Archives of Neurology* 47:1189–93, 1990.

Meier, M. J., Benton, A., Diller, L., eds. *Neuropsychological Rehabilitation.* New York: Guilford, 1987.

Mesulam, M.-M., ed. *Principles of Behavioral Neurology.* Philadelphia: Davis, 1988.

Miyamoto, M., et al. "Effects of Continuous Infusion of Cholinergic Drugs on Memory Impairment in Rats with Basal Forebrain Lesions." *Journal of Pharmacology and Experimental Therapeutics* 248:825–35, 1989.

Moore, R. G., Watts, F. N., Williams, J. "The Specificity of Personal Memories in Depression." *British Journal of Clinical Psychology* 27:275-76, 1988.

Moskowitz, H., Burns, M. "The Effects on Performance of Two Antidepressants, Alone and in Combination with Diazepam." *Progress in Neuro-Psychopharmacological and Biological Psychiatry* 12:783–92, 1988.

Nolan, K. A., et al. "A Trial of Thiamine in Alzheimer's Disease." *Archives of Neurology* 48:81–83, 1991.

Norton, N. A., et al. "Memory for Event Frequency as a Function of Depression, Age, Intentionality, and Level of Processing." *Journal of General Psychology* 115:369–81, 1988.

Quartermain, D., Judge, M., Jung, H. "Amphetamine Enhances Retrieval Following Diverse Sources of Forgetting." *Physiology and Behavior* 43:239–41, 1988.

Richardson, P. J., Wyke, M. A. "Memory Function: Effects of Different Antihypertensive Drugs." *Drugs* 35, supp. 5:80–85, 1988.

Sabin, T. D. "Dementia in the Elderly: Identifying Reversibility." *Hospital Practise*, November 30, 1986.

Sabin, T. D., Mark, V. H., eds. "Boston City Hospital Ground Rounds: A Case of Intractable Rage." *Behavioral Medicine* (July):32–41, 1981.

Sabin, T. D., Vitug, A. J., Mark, V. H. "Are Nursing Home Diagnoses and Treatment Inadequate?" *Journal of the American Medical Association* 248:321–22, 1982.

Salem, S. A., McDevitt, D. G. "Central Effects of Beta-Adrenoceptor Antagonists." *Clinical Pharmacology and Therapeutics*:52–57, 1983.

Salzman, C. *Clinical Geriatric Psychopharmacology.* New York: McGraw-Hill, 1984.

Sass, K., et al. "The Neural Substrate of Memory Impairment Demonstrated by the Intracarotid Amobarbital Procedure." *Archives of Neurology* 48:48 52, 1991.

Shealy, C., et al. "Depression: A Diagnostic, Neurochemical Profile and Therapy with Cranial Electrical Stimulation (CES)." *Journal of Neurological and Orthopaedic Medicine and Surgery* 10 (December), 1989.

———. "Therapy with Cranial Electrical Stimulation (CES)." Paper presented at the First International Conference on Stress. Montreaux, Switzerland, December 1988.

Squire, L., Butters, N. *Neuropsychology of Memory.* New York: Guilford, 1984.

Stevens, J., et al. "Deep Temporal Stimulation in Man." *Archives of Neurology* 21:157–69, 1989.

Strub, R. L., Black, F. W. *The Mental Status Examination in Neurology.* 2nd ed. Philadelphia: Davis, 1987.

Teasdale, J. D., Fogarty, S. J. "Differential Effects of Induced Mood on Retrieval of Pleasant and Unpleasant Events from Episodic Memory." *Journal of Abnormal Psychology* 88:248–57, 1979.

Turney, M. C., et al. "The NINCPS-ARDRA Work Group Criteria for the Clinical Diagnosis of Probable Alzheimer Disease." *Neurology* 38:359, 1988.

Venna, N., et al. "Reversible Depression in Binswanger's Disease." *Journal of Clinical Psychiatry* 49 (January):23–26, 1988.

Victor, M., Adams, R., Collins, G. *The Wernicke-Korsakoff Syndrome.* Philadelphia: Davis, 1989.

Vyse, S. A., Rapport, M. D. "The Effects of Methylphenidtae on Learning in Children with ADDH." *Journal of Consulting and Clinical Psychology* 57:425–35, 1989.

Wurtman, R. J., et al., eds. *Alzheimer's Disease.* Proceedings of the Fifth Meeting of the International Study Group on the Pharmacology of Memory Disorders Associated with Aging. Zurich, Switzerland, January 20–22, 1989.

Newspaper Articles

Angier, Natalie. "Gains Seen in Diagnostic Test for Alzheimer's." *New York Times,* June 6, 1990, p. A24.

Blakeslee, Sandra. "The Brain May 'See' What Eyes Cannot." *New York Times,* January 15, 1991, p. C1.

Eckholm, Erik. "Haunting Issue for U.S.: Caring for the Elderly Ill." *New York Times,* March 27, 1990, p. A1.

Kolata, Gina. "Gene Mutation That Causes Alzheimer's Is Found." *New York Times,* February 16, 1991, p. A1.

———. "The Aging Brain: The Mind Is Resilient, It's the Body That Fails." *New York Times,* April 16, 1991, p. C1.

Lewin, Tamar. "Strategies to Let Elderly Keep Some Control." *New York Times,* March 28, 1990, p. A1.

Lublin, Joann S. "Alzheimer's Linked to Aluminum in Water." *Wall Street Journal,* January 13, 1988, p. B2.

Martin, Douglas. "How to Preserve a Strong Mind: Flex It Regularly." *New York Times,* March 10, 1990, p. A27.

Waldholz, Michael. "Iron-Reducing Drug Is Found to Slow the Effects of Alzheimer's, Study Says." *Wall Street Journal,* May 31, 1991, p. B4.

Supplemental Reading

Aging and Memory

Belleville, S., Peretz, I., Malenfant, D. "Examination of the working memory components in normal aging and in dementia of the Alzheimer type." *Neuropsychologia* 34 (3):195–207, 1996.

Berg, L., McKeel, D.W., Jr., Miller, J.P., Storandt, M., Rubin, E.H., Morris, J.C., Baty, J., Coats, M., Norton, J., Goate, A.M., Price, J.L., Gearing, M., Mirra, S.S., Saunders, A.M. "Clinicopathologic studies in cognitively healthy aging and Alzheimer's disease: relation of histologic markers to dementia severity, age, sex, and apolipoprotein E genotype." *Archives of Neurology* 55 (3):326-335, 1998.

Burke, D.M., Mackay, D.G. "Memory, language, and aging." *Philosophical Transactions of the Royal Society of London — Series B: Biological Sciences* 352 (1363):1845–1856, 1997.

Cartigues, J.F., Fabrigoule, C., Leteneur, L., Amieva, H., Thiessard, F., Orgogozo, J.M. "Epidemiology of memory disorders." *Therapie,* 52 (5):503–506, 1997.

Chao, L.L., Knight, R.T. "Age-related prefrontal alterations during auditory memory." *Neurobiology of Aging* 18 (1):87–95, 1997.

Coffey, C.E., Lucke, J.R., Saxton, J.A., Ratcliff, G., Unitas, L.J., Billig, B., Bryan, R.N. "Sex differences in brain aging: a quantitative magnetic resonance imaging study." *Archives of Neurology* 55 (2):169–179, 1998.

Cullum, C.M., Filley, C.M., Kozora, E. "Episodic memory function in advanced aging and early Alzheimer's disease." *Journal of the International Neuropsychological Society* 1 (1):100–103, 1995.

Fahle, M., Daum, I. "Visual learning and memory as functions of age." *Neuropsychologia* 35 (12):1583–1589, 1997.

Harman, D. "Extending functional life span." *Experimental Gerontology* 33 (1–2):95–112, 1998.

LeMoal, S., Reymann, J.M., Thomas, V., Cattenoz, C., Lieury, A., Allain, H. "Effect of normal aging and of Alzheimer's disease on episodic memory." *Dementia and Geriatric Cognitive Disorders* 8 (5):281–287, 1997.

Masoro, E.J. "Hormesis and the antiaging action of dietary restriction." *Experimental Gerontology* 33 (1–2):61–66, 1998.

Moberg, P.J., Raz, N. "Aging and olfactory recognition memory: effect of encoding strategies and cognitive abilities." *International Journal of Neuroscience* 90 (3–4):277–291, 1997.

Palumbo, B., Parnetti, L., Nocentini, G., Cardinali, L., Brancorsini, S., Riccardi, C., Senin, U. "Apolipoprotein-E genotype in normal aging, age-associated memory impairment, Alzheimer's disease and vascular dementia patients." *Neuroscience Letters* 231 (1):59–61, 1997.

Pelosi, L., Geesken, J.M., Holly, M., Hayward, M., Blumhardt, L.D. "Working memory impairment in early multiple sclerosis. Evidence from an event related potential study of patients with clinically isolated myelopathy." *Brain* 120 (Pt II):2039–2058, 1997.

Rubin, E.H., Storandt, M., Miller, J.P., Kinscherf, D.A., Grant, E.A., Morris, J.C., Berg, L. "A prospective study of cognitive function and onset of dementia in cognitively healthy elders." *Archives of Neurology* 55 (3):395–401, 1998.

Sharps, M.J., Martin, S.S. "Spatial memory in young and older adults: environmental support and contextual influences at encoding and retrieval." *Journal of Genetic Psychology* 159 (1):5–12, 1998.

Sobreiela, T., Insausti, A., Salinas, A., Gonzalo, L.M., Insausti, R.

"The entorhinal cortex (Hippocampal formation) in aging and Alzheimer's disease. Neuroanatomical interpretation." *Revista de Medicina de la Universidad de Navarra* 41 (1):19–27, 1997.

Titov, N., Knight, R.G. "Adult age differences in controlled and automatic memory processing." *Psychology & Aging* 12 (4):565–573, 1997.

Vaupel, J.W. "The remarkable improvements in survival at older ages." *Philosophical Transactions of the Royal Society of London — Series B: Biological Sciences* 352 (1363):1799–1804, 1997.

Volkow, N.D., Gur, R.C., Wang, G.J., Fowler, J.S., Moberg, P.J., Ding, Y.S., Hitzemann, R., Smith, G., Logan, J. "Association between decline in brain dopamine activity with age and cognitive and motor impairment in healthy individuals." *American Journal of Psychiatry* 155 (3):344–349.

Weinstock, M. "Possible role of cholinergic system and disease models." *Journal of Neural Transmission. Supplementum,* 49:93–102, 1997.

Anoxia and Memory (Sleep Apnea)

Gallassi, R., Morreale, A., Montagna, P., Cortelli, P., Avoni, P., Castellani, R., Gambetti, P., Lugaresi, E. "Fatal familial insomnia: behavioral and cognitive features." *Neurology* 46 (4):935–939, 1996.

Hauri, P.J. "Cognitive deficits in insomnia patients." *Acta Neurologica Belgium* 97 (2):113–117, 1997.

Jennum, P.J., Sjol, A. "Cognitive symptoms in persons with snoring and sleep apnea. An epidemiologic study of 1,504 women and men aged 30–60 years. The Dan-MONICA II study." *Ugeskr Laeger* 157 (45):6252–6256, 1995.

Peacock, M.D., Morris, M.J., Houghland, M.A., Anders, G.T., Blanton, H.M. "Sleep apnea–hypopnea syndrome in a sample of veterans of the Persian Gulf War." *Military Medicine* 162 (4):249–251, 1997.

Perlis, M.L., Biles, D.E., Mendelson, W.B., Bootzin, R.R., Wyatt, J.K. "Psychophysiological insomnia: the behavioral model and a neurocognitive perspective." *Journal of Sleep Research* 6 (3):179–188, 1997.

Schneider-Helmert, D., Jumar, A. "Sleep, its subjective perception, and daytime performance in insomniacs with a pattern of alpha sleep." *Biological Psychiatry* 37 (2):99–105, 195.

Silver, D.A., Cross, M., Fox, B., Paxton, R.M. "Computed tomography of the brain in acute carbon monoxide poisoning." *Clinical Radiology* 51 (7):480–483, 1996.

Brain Poisoning (Street and Prescription Drugs)

Bugle, L.W. "A study of drug and alcohol use among Missouri RNs." *Journal of Psychosocial Nursing and Mental Health Services* 34 (7):41–45, 1996.

Dugurra, F. "The ethnopharmacology of hallucinogens: from 'primitive rites' to their presence on TV. Proposals for the year 2000." *Clinica Terapeutica* 147 (11):537–542, 1996.

Harding, A.J., Wong, A., Svoboda, M., Kril, J.J., Halliday, G.M. "Chronic alcohol consumption does not cause hippocampal neuron loss in humans." *Hippocampus* 7 (1):78–87, 1997.

Horowitz, B.Z. "Bromism from excessive cola consumption." *Journal of Toxicology — Clinical Toxicology* 35 (3):315–320, 1997.

Rapeli, P., Service, E., Salin, P., Holopainen, A. "A dissociation between simple and complex span impairment in alcoholics." *Memory* 5 (6):741–762, 1997.

Shimizu, K., Matsubara, K., Uezono, T., Kimura, K., Shiono, H. "Reduced dorsal hippocampal glutamate release significantly correlates with the spatial memory deficits produced by benzodiazepines and ethanol." *Neuroscience* 83 (3):701–706, 1998.

Zhang, X.L., Begleiter, H., Porjesz, B., Litke, A. "Electrophysiological evidence of memory impairment in alcoholic patients." *Biological Psychiatry* 42 (12):1157–1171, 1997.

Choline and Memory

Brambilla, F., Maggioni, M., Panerai, A.E., Sacerdote, P., Cenacchi, T. "Beta-endorphin concentration in peripheral blood mononuclear cells of elderly depressed patients — effects of phosphatidylserine therapy." *Neuropsychobiology* 34 (1):18–21, 1996.

Bruhwyler, J., Liégeois, J.R., Géczy, J. "Facilitatory effects of chronically administered citicoline on learning and memory processes in the dog." *Progress in Neuropsychopharmacological and Biological Psychiatry* 22 (1):115–128, 1998.

Furushior, M., Suzuki, S., Shishido, Y., Sakai, M., Yamatoya, H., Kudo, S., Hasimoto, S., Yokokura, T. "Effects of oral administration of soybean lecithin transphosphatidylated phosphatidylserine on impaired learning of passive avoidance in mice." *Japanese Journal of Pharmacology* 75 (4):447–450, 1997.

Masuda, Y., Kokubu, T., Yamashita, M., Ikeda, H., Inoue, S. "Egg phosphatidylcholine combined with vitamin B12 improved memory impairment following lesioning of nucleus basalis in rats." *Life Sciences* 62 (9):813–822, 1998.

Meck, W.H., Williams, C.L. "Characterization of the facilitative effects of perinatal choline supplementation on timing and temporal memory." *Neuroreport* 8 (13):2831–2835, 1997.

Spiers, P.A., Myers, D., Hochanadel, G.S., Lieberman, H.R., Wurtman, R.J. "Citicoline improves verbal memory in aging" [published erratum appears in *Archives of Neurology* 53 (10):964, 1996]. *Archives of Neurology* 53 (5):441–448, 1996.

Depression

Ackerman, D.L., Greenland, S., Bystritsky, A., Small, G.W. "Characteristics of fluoxetine versus placebo responders in a randomized trial of geriatric depression." *Psychopharmacology Bulletin* 33 (4):707–714, 1997.

Amreln, R., Stabl, M., Henauer, S., Affolter, E., Jonkanski, I. "Efficacy and tolerability of moclobemide in comparison with placebo, tricyclic antidepressants, and selective serotonin reuptake inhibitors in elderly depressed patients: a clinical overview." *Canadian Journal of Psychiatry* 42 (10):1043–1050, 1997.

Bartels, S.J., Horn, S., Sharkey, P., Levine, K. "Treatment of depression in older primary care patients in health maintenance organizations." *International Journal of Psychiatry in Medicine* 27 (3):215–231, 1997.

DasGupta, K. "Treatment of depression in elderly patients: recent advances." *Archives of Family Medicine* 7 (3):274–280, 1998.

Gareri, P., Stilo, G., Bevacqua, I., Mattace, R., Ferreri, G., DeSarro, G. "Antidepressant drugs in the elderly." *General Pharmacology* 30 (4):465–475, 1998.

Glod, C.A. "Recent advances in the pharmacotherapy of major depression." *Archives of Psychiatric Nursing* 10 (6):355–364, 1996.

Howland, R.H. "Pharmacotherapy of inpatients with bipolar depression." *Annals of Clinical Psychiatry* 9 (4):199–202, 1997.

Kasper, S. "Treatment of seasonal affective disorder (SAD) with hypericum extract." *Pharmacopsychiatry* 30 (Suppl 2):89–93, 1997.

Raffa, R.B. "Screen of receptor and uptake-site activity of hypericum component of St. John's wort reveals sigma receptor binding." *Life Sciences* 62 (16):PL265–270, 1998.

Shasha, M., Lyons, J.S., O'Mahoney, M.T., Rosenberg, A., Miller, S.I., Howard, K.I. "Serotonin reuptake inhibitors and the adequacy of antidepressant treatment." *International Journal of Psychiatry in Medicine* 27 (2):83–92, 1997.

Vorbach, E.U., Arnoldt, K.H., Hubner, W.D. "Efficacy and tolerability of St. John's wort extract LI 160 versus imipramine in patients with severe depressive episodes according to ICD-10." *Pharmacopsychiatry* 30 (Suppl 2):81–85, 1997.

Wheatley, D. "LI 160 an extract of St. John's wort, versus amitriptyline in mildly to moderately depressed outpatients — a controlled 6 week clinical trial." *Pharmacopsychiatry* 30 (Suppl 2):77–80, 1997.

Diet, Vitamins, and Memory

Bower, C., Blum, L., O'Daly, K., Higgins, C., Loutsky, F., Kosky, C. "Promotion of folate for the prevention of neural tube defects: knowledge and use of periconceptional folic acid supplements in Western Australia, 1992 to 1995." *Australian & New Zealand Journal of Public Health* 21 (7):716–721, 1997.

Easton, C.J., Bauer, L.O. "Beneficial effects of thiamine on recognition memory and P300 in abstinent cocaine-dependent patients." *Psychiatry Research* 70 (3):165–174, 1997.

Gonzalez-Burgos, I., Perez-Vega, M.I., Del Angel-Meza, A.R., Feria-Velasco, A. "Effect of tryptophan restriction on short term memory." *Physiology & Behavior* 63 (2):165–169, 1998.

Gupta, A., Moustapha, A., Jacobsen, D.W., Goormastic, M., Tuzcu, E.M., Hobbs, R., Young, J., James, K., McCarthy, P., van Lente, F., Green, R., Robinson, K. "High homocysteine, low folate, and low vitamin B6 concentrations: prevalent risk factors for vascular disease in heart transplant recipients." *Transplantation* 65 (4):544–550, 1998.

Hüppi, P.S., Schuknecht, B., Boesch, C., Bossi, E., Felblinger, J., Fusch, C., Herschkowitz, N. "Structural and neuro-behavioral delay in postnatal brain development of preterm infants." *Pediatric Research* 39 (5):895–901, 1996.

Minami, M., Kimura, S., Endo, T., Hamaue, N., Hirafugi, M., Togashi, H., Matsumoto, M., Yoshioka, M., Saito, H., Watanabe, S., Kobayashi, T., Okuyama, H. "Dietary docosahexaenoic acid increases cerebral acetylcholine levels and improves passive avoidance performance in stroke-prone spontaneously hypertensive rats." *Pharmacology, Biochemistry and Behavior* 58 (4):1123–1129, 1997.

Minami, M., Kimura, S., Endo, T., Hamaue, N., Hirafugi, M., Monma, Y., Togashi, H., Yoshioka, M., Saito, H., Watanabe, S., Kobayashi, T., Okuyama, H. "Effects of dietary docosahexaenoic acid on survival time and stroke-related behavior in stroke-prone spontaneously hypertensive rats." *General Pharmacology* 29 (3):401–407, 1997.

Soewondo, S. "The effect of iron deficiency and mental stimulation on Indonesian children's cognitive performance and development." *Kobe Journal of Medical Science* 41 (1–2):1–17, 1995.

Tanaka, M., Kariya, F., Kaihatsu, K., Nakamura, K., Asakura, T., Juroda, Y., Ohira, Y. "Effects of chronic iron deficiency anemia on brain metabolism." *Japanese Journal of Physiology* 45 (2):257–263, 1995.

Exercise and Memory

Brisswalter, J., Arcelin, R., Audiffren, M., Delignières, D. "Influence of physical exercise on simple reaction time: effect of physical fitness." *Perception and Motor Skills* 85 (3 Pt 1):1019–1027, 1997.

Féry, Y.A., Ferry, A., Vom Hofe, A., Rieu, M. "Effect of physical exhaustion on cognitive functioning." *Perception and Motor Skills* 84 (1):291–298, 1997.

Miles, C., Hardman, E. "State dependent memory produced by aerobic exercise." *Ergonomics* 41 (1):20–28, 1998.

Van Boxtel, M.P., Langerak, K., Houx, P.J., Jolles, J. "Self-reported physical activity, subjective health, and cognitive performance in older adults." *Experimental Aging Research* 22 (4):363–379, 1996.

Van Boxtel, M.P., Paas, F.G., Houx, P.J., Adam, J.J., Teeken, J.C., Jolles, J. "Aerobic capacity and cognitive performance in a cross-sectional aging study." *Medical Science, Sports and Exercise* 29 (10):1357–1365, 1997.

Hormones and Memory

Berr, C., Lafont, S., Debuire, B., Dartigues, J.R., Baulieu, E.E. "Relationships of dehydroepiandrosterone sulfate in the elderly with functional, psychological, and mental status, and short term mortality: a French community-based study." *Proceedings of National Academy of Sciences USA* 93 (23):13410–13415, 1996.

Bremner, J.D., Randall, P., Scott, T.M., Bronen, R.A., Seibyl, J.P., Southwick, S.M., Delaney, R.C., McCarthy, G., Charney, D.S., Innis, R.B. "MRI-based measurement of hippocampal volume in patients with combat-related posttraumatic stress disorder." *American Journal of Psychiatry* 152 (7):973–981, 1995.

Frye, C.A., Sturgis, J.D. "Neurosteroids affect spatial/reference, working, and long-term memory of female rats." *Neurobiology, Learning and Memory* 64 (1):83–96, 195.

Kirschbaum, C., Wolf, O.T., May, M., Wippich, W., Hellhammer,

D.H. "Stress- and treatment-induced elevations of cortisol levels associated with impaired declarative memory in healthy adults." *Life Sciences* 58 (17):1475–1483, 1996.

Lupien, S.J., Gaudreau, S., Tchiteya, B.M., Maheu, F., Sharma, S., Nair, N.P., Hauger, R.L., McEwen, B.S., Meaney, M.J. "Stress-induced declarative memory impairment in healthy elderly subjects: relationship to cortisol reactivity." *Journal of Clinical Endrocrinological Metabolism* 82 (7):2070–2075, 1997.

O'Brien, J.T., Ames, D., Schweitzer, I., Colman, P., Desmond, P., Tress, B. "Clinical and magnetic resonance imaging correlates of hypothalamic-pituitary-adrenal axis function in depression and Alzheimer's disease." *British Journal of Psychiatry* 168 (6):679–687, 1996.

Seeman, T.E., McEwen, B.S., Singer, B.H., Albert, M.S., Rowe, J.W. "Increase in urinary cortisol excretion and memory declines: MacArthur studies of successful aging." *Journal of Clinical Endocrinological Metabolism* 82 (8):2458–2465, 1997.

Wolf, O.T., Neumann, O., Hellhammer, D.H., Geiben, A.C., Strasburger, C.J., Dressendörfer, R.A., Pirke, K.M., Kirschbaum, C. "Effects of a two-week physiological dehydroepiandrosterone substitution on cognitive performance and well-being in healthy elderly women and men." *Journal of Clinical Endocrinological Metabolism* 82 (7):2363–2367, 1997.

Wolf, O.T., Koster, B., Kirschbaum, C., Pietrowsky, R., Kern, W., Hellhammer, D.H., Born, J., Fehm, H.L. "A single administration of dehydroepiandrosterone does not enhance memory performance in young healthy adults, but immediately reduces cortisol levels." *Biological Psychiatry* 42 (9):845–848, 1997.

Wolkowitz, O.M., Reus, V.I., Roberts, E., Manfredi, F., Chan, T., Raum, W.J., Ormiston, S., Johnson, R., Canick, J., Brizendine, L., Weingartner, H. "Dehydroepiandrosterone (DHEA) treatment of depression." *Biological Psychiatry* 41 (3):311–318, 1997.

Yanase, T., Fukahori, M., Taniguchi, S., Nishi, Y., Sakai, Y., Takayanagi, R., Haji, M., Nawata, H. "Serum dehydroepiandrosterone (DHEA) and DHEA-sulfate (DHEA-S) in

Alzheimer's disease and in cerebrovascular dementia." *Endocrinology Journal* 43 (1):119–123, 1996.

Memory Classification

Athanassopoulou, A., Gouliamos, A., Papageorgiou, C. "Cognitive function in non-demented individuals complaining of short term memory disturbances: a study with event related potential (P300) and brain CT scan." *Electromyography and Clinical Neurophysiology* 37 (5):317–320, 1997.

Allain, H., Lieury, A., Quemener, V., Thomas, V., Reymann, J.M., Gandon, J.M. "Procedural memory and Parkinson's disease." *Dementia* 6 (3):174–178, 1995.

Bodner, M., Zhou, Y.D., Shaw, G.L., Fuster, J.M. "Symmetric temporal patterns in cortical spike trains during performance of a short term memory task." *Neurological Research* 19 (5):509–514, 1997.

Buckner, R.L., Koutstall, W. "Functional neuroimaging studies of encoding, priming, and explicit memory retrieval. [Review]." *Proceedings of the National Academy of Sciences of the United States of America* 95 (3):891–898, 1998.

Carlson, S., Rama, P., Artchakov, D., Linnankoski, I. "Effects of music and white noise on working memory performance in monkeys." *Neuroreport* 8 (13):2853–2856, 1997.

Cipolotti, L., Warrington, E.K. "Semantic memory and reading abilities: a case report." *Journal of the International Neuropsychological Society* 1 (1):104–110, 1995.

Cohen, J.D., Perlstein, W.M., Braver, T.S., Nystrom, L.E., Noll, D.C., Nonides, J., Smith, E.E. "Temporal dynamics of brain activation during a working memory task." *Nature* 386 (6625):604–608, 1997.

Curran, T., Hintzman, D.L. "Violations of the independence assumption in process dissociation." *Journal of Experimental Psychology: Learning, Memory, & Cognition* 21 (3):531–547, 1995.

Fiez, J.A., Faife, E.A., Balota, D.A., Schwarz, J.P., Raichle, M.E., Petersen, S.E. "A positron emission tomography study of the short term maintenance of verbal information." *Journal of Neuroscience* 16 (2):808–822, 1996.

Herlitz, A., Nilsson, L.G., Backman, L. "Gender differences in episodic memory." *Memory & Cognition* 25 (6):801–811, 1997.

Isaki, E., Plante, E. "Short term and working memory differences in language/learning disabled and normal adults." *Journal of Communicative Disorders* 30 (6):427–436, quiz 436–37, 1997.

Kamiya, S. "The influence of an emotion on the retention of episodic scenes." *Shinrigaku Kenkyu, Japanese Journal of Psychology* 68 (4):290–297, 1997.

Klingberg, T., O'Sullivan, B.T., Roland, P.E. "Bilateral activation of frontoparietal networks by incrementing demand in a working memory task." *Cerebral Cortex* 7 (5):465–471, 1997.

Lambon, Ralph M.A., Patterson, K., Hodges, J.R. "The relationship between naming and semantic knowledge for different categories in dementia of Alzheimer's type." *Neuropsychologia* 35 (9):1251–1260, 1997.

Martin-Loeches, M., Rubia, F.J. "Encoding into working memory of spatial location, color, and shape: electrophysiological investigations." *International Journal of Neuroscience* 91 (3–4):277–294, 1997.

McCarthy, G., Puce, A., Constable, R.T., Krystal, J.H., Gore, J.C., Goldman-Rakic, P. "Activation of human prefrontal cortex during spatial and nonspatial working memory tasks measured by functional MRI." *Cerebral Cortex* 6 (4):600–611, 1996.

McIntosh, A.R., Grady, C.L., Haxby, J.V., Ungerleider, L.G., Horwitz, B. "Changes in limbic and prefrontal functional interactions in a working memory task for faces." *Cerebral Cortex* 6 (4):571–584, 1996.

Nyberg, L., McIntosh, A.R., Tulving, E. "Functional brain imaging of episodic and semantic memory with positron emission tomography. [Review] [60 refs]." *Journal of Molecular Medicine* 76 (1):48–53, 1998.

Parkin, A.J. "Human memory: novelty, association and the brain. [Review] [7 refs]." *Current Biology* 7 (12):R768–769, 1997.

Poldrack, R.A., Gabrieli, J.D. "Functional anatomy of long-term memory. [Review] [160 refs]." *Journal of Clinical Neurophysiology* 14 (4):294–310, 1997.

Rassin, E., Merckelbach, H., Muris, P. "Effects of thought suppression on episodic memory." *Behaviour Research & Therapy* 35 (11):1035–1038, 1997.

Robbins, T.W. "Refining the taxonomy of memory." *Science* 273 (5280):1353–1354, 1996.

Ruchkin, D.S., Johnson, R., Jr., Grafman, J., Canoune, H., Ritter, W. "Multiple visuospatial working memory buffers: evidence from spatiotemporal patterns of brain activity" [published erratum appears in *Neuropsychologia* 35 (4):572, 1997]. *Neuropsychologia* 35 (2):195–209, 1997.

Schimmack, U., Hartmann, K. "Individual differences in the memory representation of emotional episodes: exploring the cognitive processes in repression." *Journal of Personality & Social Psychology* 73 (5):1064–1079, 1997.

Schmitter-Edgecombe, M. "The effects of divided attention on implicit and explicit memory performance." *Journal of the International Neuropsychological Society* 2 (2):111–125, 1996.

Schrijnemakers, J.M., Raaijmakers, J.G. "Adding new word associations to semantic memory: evidence for two interactive learning components." *Acta Psychologica* 96 (1–2):103–132, 1997.

Smith, E.E., Jonides, J., Marshuetz, C., Koeppe, R.A. "Components of verbal working memory: evidence from neuroimaging. [Review] [32 refs]." *Proceedings of the National Academy of Sciences of the United States of America* 95 (3):876–882, 1998.

Verfaellie, M., Reiss, L., Roth, H.L. "Knowledge of New English vocabulary in amnesia: an examination of premorbidly acquired semantic memory." *Journal of the International Neuropsychological Society* 1 (5):443–453, 1995.

Wheeler, M.A., Stuss, D.T., Tulving, E. "Frontal lobe damage produces episodic memory impairment." *Journal of the International Neuropsychological Society* 1 (6):525–536, 1995.

Wong, C.W. "Two circuits to convert short term memory into long term memory. [Review] [52 refs]." *Medical Hypotheses* 49 (5):375–378, 1997.

Memory Localization
(Functional MRI and PET)

Berthoz, A. "Parietal and hippocampal contribution to topokinetic and topographic memory [Review] [94 refs]." *Philosophical Transactions of the Royal Society of London — Series B: Biological Sciences* 352 (1360):1437–1448, 1997.

Blaxton, T.A., Bookheimer, S.Y., Zeffiro, T.A., Figlozzi, C.M., Gaillard, W.D., Theodore, W.H. "Functional mapping of human memory using PET: comparisons of conceptual and perceptual tasks." *Canadian Journal of Experimental Psychology* 50 (1):42–56, 1996.

Bogner, P., Berenyi, E., Kover, G., Petrasi, Z., Repa, I. "[Principals of functional MRI imaging and its possibilities in the study of cerebral cortex activation] [Review] [38 refs] [Hungarian]." *Orvosi Hetilap* 138 (38):2391–2395, 1997.

Coull, J.T., Frith, C.D., Frackowiak, R.S., Grasby, P.M. "A frontoparietal network for rapid visual information processing: a PET study of sustained attention and working memory." *Neuropsychologia* 34 (11):1085–1095, 1996.

Courtney, S.M., Ungerleider, L.G., Keil, K., Haxby, J.V. "Transient and sustained activity in a distributed neural system for human memory." *Nature* 386 (6625):608–611, 1997.

Eustache, F., Desgranges, B., Petit-Taboue, M.C., de la Sayette, V., Piot, V., Sable, C., Marchal, G., Baron, J.C. "Transient global amnesia: implicit/explicit memory dissociation and PET assessment of brain perfusion and oxygen metabolism in the acute stage. [Review] [90 refs]." *Journal of Neurology, Neurosurgery & Psychiatry* 63 (3):357–367, 1997.

Evans, J., Wilson, B., Wraight, E.P., Hodges, J.R. "Neuropsychological and SPECT scan findings during and after transient global amnesia: evidence for the differential impairment of remote episodic memory." *Journal of Neurology, Neurosurgery & Psychiatry* 56 (11):1227–1230, 1993.

Fernandez, G., Weyerts, H., Schrader-Bolsche, M., Tendolkar, I.,

Smid, H.G., Tempelmann, C., Hinirichs, H., Scheich, H., Elger, C.E., Mangun, G.R., Heinze, H.J. "Successful verbal encoding into episodic memory engages the posterior hippocampus: a parametrically analyzed functional magnetic resonance imaging study." *Journal of Neuroscience* 18 (5):1841–1847, 1998.

Fletcher, P.C., Dolan, R.J., Shallice, T., Firth, C.D., Frackowiak, R.S., Friston, K.J. "Is multivariate analysis of PET data more revealing than the univariate approach? Evidence from a study of episodic memory retrieval." *Neuroimage* 3 (3 Pt 1):209–215, 1996.

Friedland, R.P. "Brain imaging in dementia." *Mediguide to Geriatric Neurology* 1 (4):1–8, 1998.

Grossman, M., Payer, F., Onishi, K., White-Devine, T., Morrison, D., D'Esposito, M., Robinson, K., Alavi, A. "Constraints on the cerebral basis for semantic processing from neuroimaging studies of Alzheimer's disease." *Journal of Neurology, Neurosurgery & Psychiatry* 63 (2):152–158, 1997.

Kapur, S., Craik, F.I., Jones, C., Brown, G.M., Houle, S., Tulving, E. "Functional role of the prefrontal cortex in retrieval of memories: a PET study." *Neuroreport* 6 (14):1880–1884, 1995.

Kim, S.G., Tsekos, N.V., Ashe, J. "Multi-slice perfusion-based functional MRI using the FAIR technique: comparison of CBF and BOLD effects." *New Medical Research in Biomedicine* 10 (4–5):191–196, 1997.

Kopelman, M.D., Stanhope, N., Kingsley, D. "Temporal and spatial context memory in patients with focal frontal, temporal lobe, and diencephalic lesions." *Neuropsychologia* 35 (12):1533–1545, 1997.

Le, T.H., Hu, X. "Methods for assessing accuracy and reliability in functional MRI." *New Medical Research in Biomedicine* 10 (4–5):160–164, 1997.

Maguire, E.A. "Hippocampal involvement in human topographical memory: evidence from functional imaging. [Review] [34 refs]." *Philosophical Transactions of the Royal Society of London — Series B: Biological Sciences* 352 (1360):1475–1480, 1997.

Markowitsch, H.J., Calacrese, P., Wiurker, M., Durwen, H.F., Kessler, J., Babinsky, R., Brechtelsbauer, D., Heuser, L., Gehlen, W. "The amygdala's contribution to memory — a study on two patients with Urbach-Wiethe disease." *Neuroreport* 5 (11):1349–1352, 1994.

McCarthy, G., Puce, A., Constable, R.T., Krystal, J.H., Gore, J.C., Goldman-Rakic, P. "Activation of human prefrontal cortex during spatial and nonspatial working memory tasks measured by functional MRI." *Cerebral Cortex* 7 (4):600–611, 1996.

Mellers, J.D., Bullmore, E., Brammer, M., Williams, S.C., Andrew, C., Sachs, N., Andrews, C., Cox, T.S., Simmons, A., Woodruf, P., *et al.* "Neural correlates of working memory in a visual letter monitoring task: an fMRI study." *Neuroreport* 8 (1):109–112, 1995.

Miceli, G., Colosimo, C., Daniele, A., Marra, C., Perani, D., Fazio, F. "Isolated amnesia with slow onset and stable course, without ensuing dementia: MRI and PET data and a six-year neuropsychological follow-up." *Dementia* 7 (2):104–110, 1996.

Milner, B., Johnsrude, I., Crane, J. "Right medial temporal lobe contribution to object location memory." *Philosophical Transactions of the Royal Society of London — Series B: Biological Sciences* 352 (1360):1469–1474, 1997.

Nyberg, L., McIntosh, A.R., Tulving, E. "Functional brain imaging of episodic and semantic memory with positron emission tomography. [Review] [60 refs]." *Journal of Molecular Medicine* 76 (1):48–53, 1998.

Schacter, D.L., Uecker, A., Reiman, E., Yun, L.S., Bandy, D., Chen, K., Cooper, L.A., Curran, T. "Effects of size and orientation change on hippocampal activation during episodic recognition: a PET study." *Neuroreport* 8 (18):393–398, 1997.

Schlosser, R., Hutchinson, M., Joseffer, S., Rusinek, H., Saarimaki, A., Stevenson, J., Dewey, S.L., Brodie, J.D. "Functional magnetic resonance imaging of human brain activity in a verbal fluency task." *Journal of Neurology, Neurosurgery & Psychiatry* 64 (4):492–498, 1998.

Memory Testing

Buschke, H., Shilwinski, M.J., Kuslansky, G., Lipton, R.B. "Diagnosis of early dementia by the Double Memory Test: encoding specificity improves diagnostic sensitivity and specificity." *Neurology* 48 (4):989–997, 1997.

Frank, Y., Seiden, J., Napolitano, B. "Visual event related potentials and reaction time in normal adults, normal children, and children with attention deficit hyperactivity disorder: differences in short term memory processing." *International Journal of Neuroscience* 88 (1–2):109–124, 1996.

Gfeller, J.D., Horn, G.J. "The East Boston Memory Test: a clinical screening measure for memory impairment in the elderly." *Journal of Clinical Psychology* 52 (2):191–196, 1996.

Hall, S., Pinkston, S.L., Szalda-Petree, A.C., Coronis, A.R. "The performance of healthy older adults on the Continuous Visual Memory Test and the Visual-Motor Integration Test: preliminary findings." *Journal of Clinical Psychology* 52 (4):449–454, 1996.

Hon, J., Huppert, F.A., Holland, A.J., Watson, P. "The value of the Rivermead Behavioral Memory Test (Children's Version) in an epidemiological study of older adults with Down Syndrome." *British Journal of Clinical Psychology* 37 (Pt 1):15–29, 1998.

Kazmerski, V.A., Friedman, D. "Effects of multiple presentations of words on event-related potential and reaction time repetition effects in Alzheimer's patients and young and older controls." *Neuropsychiatry, Neuropsychology and Behavioral Neurology* 10 (1):32–47, 1997.

Luciana, M., Nelson, C.A. "The functional emergence of prefrontally-guided working memory systems in four to eight year old children." *Neuropsychologia* 36 (3):273–293, 1998.

Magnussen, S., Idas, E., Myhre, S.H. "Representation of orientation and spatial frequency in perception and memory: a choice reaction-time analysis." *Journal of Experimental Psychology, Human Perception and Performance* 24 (3):707–718, 1998.

Nettelbeck, T., Rabbitt, P.M., Wilson, C., Batt, R. "Uncoupling learning from initial recall: the relationship between speech and memory deficits in old age." *British Journal of Psychology* 87 (Pt 4):593–607, 1996.

Nielsen, U., Dahl, R., White, R.F., Grandjean, P. "Computer assisted neuropsychological testing of children." *Ugeskrift for Laeger* 160 (24):3557–3561, 1998.

Palmer, D.L., Folds-Bennett, T. "Performance on two attention tasks as a function of sex and competition." *Perceptual & Motor Skills* 86 (2):363–370, 1998.

Parker, E.S., Eaton, E.M., Whipple, S.C., Heseltine, P.N., Bridge, T.P. "University of Southern California Repeatable Episodic Memory Test." *Journal of Clinical Experimental Neuropsychology* 17 (6):926–936, 1995.

Robinson, M.D., Johnson, J.T., Herndon, F. "Reaction time and assessments of cognitive effort as predictors of eyewitness memory accuracy and confidence." *Journal of Applied Psychology* 82 (3):416–425, 1997.

Salthouse, T.A., Becker, J.T. "Independent effects of Alzheimer's disease on neuropsychological functioning." *Neuropsychology* 12 (2):242–252, 1998.

Schagen, S., Schmand, B., deSterke, S., Lindeboom, J. "Amsterdam Short-Term Memory test: a new procedure for the detection of feigned memory deficits." *Journal of Clinical Experimental Neuropsychology* 19 (1):43–51, 1997.

Schwartz, M.L., Carruth, F., Binns, M.A., Brandys, C., Moulton, R., Snow, W.G., Stuss, D.T. "The course of posttraumatic amnesia: three little words." *Canadian Journal of Neurological Sciences* 25 (2):108–116, 1998.

Pain and Memory

Cain, C.K., Francis, J.M., Plone, M.A., Emerich, D.F., Lindner, M.D. "Pain related disability and effects of chronic morphine in the adjuvant-induced arthritis model of chronic pain." *Physiology and Behavior* 62 (1):199–205, 197.

Capuzzo, M., Bianconi, M., Contu, P., Cingolani, E., Verri, M., Gritti, G. "Memory for postoperative pain six months after discharge from the hospital." *Minerva Anestesiol* 63 (1–2):39–45, 1997.

Christenfeld, N. "Memory for pain and the delayed effects of distraction." *Health and Psychology* 16 (4):327–330, 1997.

Coghill, R.C., Sang, C.N., Berman, K.F., Bennett, G.J., Iadarola, M. "Global cerebral blood flow decreases during pain." *Journal of Cerebral Blood Flow & Metabolism* 18 (2):141–147, 1998.

Iadarola, M., Max, M.G., Berman, K.F., Byas-Smith, M.G., Coghill, R.C., Gracely, R.H., Bennett, G.J. "Unilateral decrease in thalamic activity observed with positron emission tomography in patients with chronic neuropathic pain." *Pain* 63 (1):55–64, 1995.

Overchkin, A.M., Kujushkin, M.L., Gnezdilov, A.V., Reshetniak, V.K. "Adequacy of amputation analgesia as a factor preventing the triggering of pain memory in the genesis of phantom pain syndrome." *Anesteziol Reanimatol* (2):56–59, 1995.

Schnurr, R.F., MacDonald, M.R. "Memory complaints in chronic pain." *Clinical Journal of Pain* 11 (2):103–111, 1995.

Parkinson's Disease

Lang, A.E., Lozano, A.M. "Parkinson's Disease, first of two parts." *New England Journal of Medicine* 339 (15):1044–1053, 1998.

Prevention of Alzheimer's Disease

Aisen, P.S., Pasinetti, G.M. "Glucocorticoids in Alzheimer's disease: The story so far." *Drugs and Aging* 12 (1):1–6, 1998.

Anderer, P., Saletu, B., Semlitsch, H.V., Pascual-Marqui, R.D. "Electrical sources of P300 event-related brain potentials revealed by low resolution electromagnetic tomography. 2. Effects of nootropic therapy in age associated memory impairment." *Neuropsychobiology* 37 (1):28–35, 1998.

Blom, M.A., van Twillert, M.G., deVries, S.C., Engels, F., Finch, C.E., Veerhuis, R., Eikelenboom, P. "NSAIDS inhibit the IL-1 beta-induced IL-6 release from human post-mortem astrocytes: the involvement of prostaglandin E2." *Brain Research* 777 (1–2):210–218, 1997.

Cohen-Salmon, C., Venault, P., Martin, B., Raffalli-Sebille, M.J., Barkats, M., Clostre, F., Pardon, M.C., Christen, Y., Chapouthier, G. "Effects of Gingko biloba extract (Egb761) on learning and possible actions on aging." *Journal of Physiology* (Paris) 91 (6):291-300, 1997.

Fink, G., Sumner, B.E., Rosie, R., Grace, O., Quinn, J.P. "Estrogen control of central neurotransmission: effect on mood, mental state, and memory." *Cellular Molecular Neurobiology* 16 (3):325–344, 1996.

Flood, J.F., Morley, J.E., Roberts, E. "Pregnenolone sulfate enhances post training memory processes when injected in very low doses into limbic system structures: the amygdala is by far the most sensitive." *Proceedings of National Academy of Sciences USA* 92 (3):10806–10810, 1995.

Garg, R.K., Nag, D., Agrawal, A. "A double blind placebo controlled trial of gingko biloba extract in acute cerebral ischemia." *Journal of Associated Physicians of India* 43 (11):760–763, 1995.

Haase, J., Halama, P., Horr, R. "Effectiveness of brief infusions with Ginkgo biloba Special Extract Egb 761 in dementia of the vascular and Alzheimer type." *Gerontology and Geriatrics* 29 (4):302–309, 1996.

Ingvar, M., Ambros-Ingerson, J., Davis, M., Granger, R., Kessler, M., Rogers, G.A., Schehr, R.S., Lynch, G. "Enhancement by an ampakine of memory encoding in humans." *Experimental Neurology* 146 (2):553–559, 197.

Kanowski, S., Herrmann, W.M., Stephan, K., Wierich, W., Horr, R. "Proof of efficacy of the ginkgo biloba special extract Egb 761 in outpatients suffering from mild to moderate primary degenerative dementia of the Alzheimer type or multi-infarct dementia." *Pharmacopsychiatry* 29 (2):47–56, 1996.

Lerner, A., Koss, E., Debanne, S., Rowland, D., Smyth, K., Friedland, R. "Smoking and oestrogen-replacement therapy as protective factors for Alzheimer's disease." *Lancet* 349 (9049):403–404, 1997.

Marchilhac, A., Dakine, N., Burhim, N., Guillaume, V., Grino, M., Drieu, K., Oliver, C. "Effect of chronic administration of

Ginkgo biloba extract to Ginkglide on the hypothalamic-pituitary-adrenal axis in the rat." *Life Sciences* 62 (25):2329–2340, 1998.

Maurer, K., Ihl, R., Dierks, T., Frolich, L. "Clinical efficacy of Ginkgo biloba special extract Egb 761 in dementia of the Alzheimer type." *Journal of Psychiatric Research* 31 (6):645–655, 1997.

Michaelis, M.L., Ranciat, N., Chen, Y., Bechtel, M., Ragan, R., Hepperle, M., Liu, Y., Georg, G. "Protection against beta-amyloid toxicity in primary neurons by paclitaxel (Taxol)." *Journal of Neurochemistry* 70 (4):1623–1627, 1998.

Packard, M.G., Teather, L.A. "Intra-hippocampal estradiol infusion enhances memory in ovariectomized rats." *Neuroreport* 8 (14):3009–3013, 1997.

Parks, R.W., Becker, R.E., Rippey, R.F., Gilbert, D.G., Matthew, J.R., Kabatay, E., Young, C.S., Vohs, C., Danz, V., Keim, P., Collins, G.T., Zigler, S.S., Urycki, P.G. "Increased regional cerebral glucose metabolism and semantic memory performance in Alzheimer's disease: a pilot double blind transdermal nicotine positron emission tomography study." *Neuropsychology Review* 6 (2):61–79, 1996.

Sastre, J., Millan, A., Garcia de la Asuncion, J., Pla, R., Juan, G., Pallard, O., O'Connor, E., Martin, J.A., Droy-Lefaix, M.T., Vina, J. "A Gingko biloba extract (Egb 761) prevents mitochondrial aging by protecting against oxidative stress." *Free Radical Biological Medicine* 24 (2):298–304, 1998.

Sharma, A., Parikh, V., Singh, M. "Pharmacological basis of drug therapy of Alzheimer's disease." *Indian Journal of Experimental Biology* 35 (11):1146–1155, 1997.

Sherwin, B.B. "Estrogen effects on cognition in menopausal women." *Neurology* 48 (5 Suppl 7):S21–26, 1997.

Socci, D.J., Sanberg, P.R., Arendash, G.W. "Nicotine enhances Morris water maze performance of young and aged rats." *Neurobiology of Aging* 16 (5):857–860, 1995.

Tomaz, C., Nogueira, P.J. "Facilitation of memory by peripheral administration of substance P." *Behavioral Brain Research* 83 (1–2):143–145, 1997.

Wesnes, K.A., Faleni, R.A., Hefting, N.R., Hoogsteen, G., Houben, J.J., Jenkins, E., Jonkman, J.H., Leonard, J., Petrini, O., van Lier, J.J. "The cognitive, subjective, and physical effects of a ginkgo biloba/panax ginseng combination in healthy volunteers with neurasthenic complaints." *Psychopharmacology Bulletin* 33 (4):677–683, 1997.

Stress, Brain Injury, and Memory

Hershey, T., Craft, S., Bhargava, N., White, N.H. "Memory and insulin dependent diabetes mellitus (IDDM); effects of childhood onset and severe hypoglycemia." *Journal of International Neuropsychological Society* 3 (6):509–520, 1997.

Jenkins, M.A., Langlais, P.J., Delis, D., Cohen, R. "Learning and memory in rape victims with posttraumatic stress disorder." *American Journal of Psychiatry* 155 (2):278–279, 1998.

Laurent, B., Van der Linden, M., Ali Cherif, A., Hibert, O., Truche, A. "Rehabilitation of memory: strategies, indications and limits." *Therapie* 52 (5):509–513, 1997.

Lundh, L.G., Czyzkow, S., Ost, L.G. "Explicit and implicit memory bias in panic disorder with agoraphobia." *Behaviour Research & Therapy* 35 (11):1003–1014, 1997.

Papagno, C., Baddeley, A. "Confabulation in dysexecutive patient; implication for models of retrieval." *Cortex* 33 (4):743–752, 1997.

Pope, K.S. "Memory, abuse and science. Questioning claims about the false memory syndrome epidemic [Review] [140 refs]" [published erratum appears in *American Psychology* 52 (9):106, 1997]. *American Psychology* 51 (9):957–974, 1996.

Pratt, P., Tallis, F., Eysenck, M. "Information-processing, storage characteristics and worry." *Behaviour Research & Therapy* 35 (11):1015–1023, 1997.

Suhr, J., Tranel, D., Wefel, J., Barrash, J. "Memory performance after head injury: contributions of malingering, litigation status, psychological factors, and medication use." *Journal of Clinical Experimental Neuropsychology* 19 (4):500–514, 1997.

Tate, R.L. "Beyond one-bun, two-shoe; recent advances in the psychological rehabilitation of memory disorders after acquired brain injury. [Review] [62 refs]." *Brain Injury* 11 (12):907–918, 1997.

Vasterling, J.J., Brailey, K., Constans, J.I., Sutker, P.B. "Attention and memory dysfunction in posttraumatic stress disorder." *Neuropsychology* 12 (1):125–133, 1998.

Stroke Prevention and Treatment

Abbott, R.D., Curb, J.D., Rodriguez, B.L., Sharp, D.S., Burchfiel, C.M., Yano, K. "Effects of dietary calcium and milk consumption on risk of thromboembolic stroke in older middle-aged men. The Honolulu Heart Program." *Stroke* 27 (5):813–818, 1996.

Abyad, A., Kligman, E. "Primary polycythaemia vera in the elderly." *Journal of International Medical Research* 22 (2):121–129, 1994.

Alexander, M.P. "Specific semantic memory loss after hypoxic-ischemic injury." *Neurology* 48 (1):165–173, 1997.

Cappuccio, F.P., Markandu, N.D., Carney, C., Sagnella, G.A., Mac-Gregor, G.A. "Double-blind randomized trial of modest salt restriction in older people." *Lancet* 350 (9081):850–854, 1997.

Daviglus, M.L., Orencia, A.J., Dyer, A.R., Liu, K., Morris, D.K., Persky, V., Chavez, N., Goldberg, J., Drum, M., Shekelle, R.B., Stamler, J. "Dietary vitamin C, beta-carotene and 30 year risk of stroke: results from the Western Electric Study." *Neuroepidemiology* 16 (2):69–77, 1997.

DeDevn, P.P., Reuck, J.D., Deberdt, W., Vlietinck, R., Orgogozo, J.M. "Treatment of acute ischemic stroke with piracetam. Members of the Piracetam in Acute Stroke Study (PASS) Group." *Stroke* 28 (12):2347–2352, 1997.

de la Torre, J.C., Nelson, N., Sutherland, R.J., Pappas, B.A. "Reversal of ischemic-induced chronic memory dysfunction in aging rats with free radical scavenger-glycolytic intermediate combination." *Brain Research* 779 (1–2):285–288, 1998.

Demrow, H.S., Slane, P.R., Folts, J.D. "Administration of wine and grape juice inhibits in vivo platelet activity and thrombosis in stenosed canine coronary arteries." *Circulation* 91 (4):1182–1188, 1995.

Gale, C.R., Martyn, C.N., Winger, P.D., Cooper, C. "Vitamin C and risk of death from stroke and coronary heart disease in cohort of elderly people." *British Medical Journal* 310 (6994):1563–1566, 1995.

Giles, W.H., Kittner, S.J., Anda, R.F., Croft, J.B., Casper, M.L. "Serum folate and risk for ischemic stroke. First National Health and Nutrition Examination Survey epidemiologic follow-up study." *Stroke* 26 (7):1166–1170, 1995.

Gillman, M.W., Cupples, L.A., Gagnon, D., Posner, B.M., Ellison, R.C., Castelli, W.P., Wolf, P.A. "Protective effect of fruits and vegetables on development of stroke in men." *Journal of American Medical Association* 273 (24):1113–1117, 1995.

Gillman, M.W., Cupples, L.A., Millen, B.E., Ellison, R.C., Wolf, P.A. "Inverse association of dietary fat with development of ischemic stroke in men." *Journal of American Medical Association* 278 (24):2145–2150, 1997.

Hansagi, H., Romelsjö, A., Gerhardsson de Verdier, M., Andréasson, S., Leifman, A. "Alcohol consumption and stroke mortality. 20 year follow-up of 15,077 men and women." *Stroke* 26 (10):1768–1773, 1995.

Hu, F.B., Stampfer, M.J., Manson, J.E., Rimm, E., Colditz, G.A., Rosner, B.A., Hennekens, C.H., Willett, W.C. "Dietary fat intake and the risk of coronary heart disease in women." *New England Journal of Medicine* 337 (21):1491–1499, 1997.

Keli, S.O., Hertog, M.G., Feskens, E.J., Fromhout, D. "Dietary flavonoids, antioxidant vitamins, and incidence of stroke: the Zutphen study." *Archives of Internal Medicine* 156 (6):637–642, 1996.

Kiss, B., Karpati, E. "Mechanism of action of vinpocetine." *Acta Pharmaceutica Hungarica* 66 (5):213–224, 1996.

Kiyohara, Y., Kato, I., Iwamoto, H., Nakayama, K., Fujishima, M. "The impact of alcohol and hypertension on stroke incidence in a general Japanese population. The Hisayama Study." *Stroke* 26 (3):368–372, 1995.

Mancini, M., Parfitt, V.J., Rubba, P. "Antioxidants in the Mediterranean diet." *Canadian Journal of Cardiology* 11 (Suppl G):105G–109G, 1995.

Supplemental Reading

Mark, S.D., Wang, W., Fraumeni, J.F., Jr., Li, J.Y., Taylor, P.R., Wang, G.Q., Dawsey, S.M., Li, B., Blot, W.J. "Do nutritional supplements lower the risk of stroke or hypertension?" *Epidemiology* 9 (1):9–15, 1998.

Miyazaki, M. "The effect of a cerebral vasodilator, vinpocetine, on cerebral vascular resistance evaluated by the Doppler ultrasonic technique in patients with cerebrovascular diseases." *Angiology* 46 (1):53–58, 1995.

Morris, M.C., Manson, J.E., Rosner, B., Buring, J.E., Eillett, W.C., Hennekens, C.H. "Fish consumption and cardiovascular disease in the physicians' health study: a prospective study." *American Journal of Epidemiology* 142 (2):166–175, 1995.

Murakami, Y., Tanaka, E., Sakai, Y., Matsumoto, K., Li, H.B., Watanabe, H. "Tacrine improves working memory deficit caused by permanent occlusions of bilateral common carotid arteries in rats." *Japanese Journal of Pharmacology* 75 (4):443–446, 1997.

Ness, A.R., Powles, J.W., Khaw, K.T. "Vitamin C and cardiovascular disease: a systematic review." *Journal of Cardiovascular Risk* 3 (6):513–521, 1996.

Nunn, J., Hodges, H. "Cognitive deficits induced by global cerebral ischemia: relationship to brain damage and reversal by transplants." *Behavioural Brain Research* 65 (1):1–31, 1994.

Orencia, A.J., Daviglus, M.L., Dyer, A.R., Shekelle, R.B., Stamler, J. "Fish consumption and stroke in men. 30-year findings of the Chicago Western Electric Study." *Stroke* 27 (2):204–209, 1996.

Paroczai, M., Kiss, B., Karpati, E. "Effect of RGH-2716 on learning and memory deficits of young and aged rats in water-labyrinth." *Brain Research Bulletin* 45 (5):475–488, 1998.

Perry, I.J., Refsum, H., Morris, R.W., Ebrahim, S.B., Ueland, P.M., Shaper, A.G. "Prospective study of serum total homocystene concentration and risk of stroke in middle aged British men." *Lancet* 346 (8987):1395–1398, 1995.

Ricci, S., Celani, M.G., Righetti, E., Caruso, A., DeMedio, G., Trovarelli, G., Romoli, S., Stragliotto, E., Spizzichino, L.

"Fatty acid dietary intake and the risk of ischemic stroke: a multicentre case-controlled study. UFA Study Group." *Journal of Neurology* 244 (6):360–364, 1997.

Rice, R. "Fish and healthy pregnancy: more than just a red herring!" *Professional Care of Mother and Child* 6 (6):171–173, 1996.

Robinson, K., Arheart, K., Refsum, H., Brattstrom, L., Boers, G., Ueland, P., Rubba, P., Palma-Reis, R., Meleady, R., Daly, L., Witteman, J., Graham, I. "Low circulating folate and vitamin B6 concentrations: risk factors for stroke, peripheral vascular disease, and coronary artery disease. European COMAC Group." *Circulation* 97 (5):437–443, 1998.

Salonen, J.R., Seepänen, K., Nyyssönen, K., Korpela, H., Kauhanen, J., Kantola, M., Tuomilehto, J., Esterbauer, H., Tatzber, F., Salonen, R. "Intake of mercury from fish, lipid peroxidatin, and the risk of myocardial infarction and coronary, cardiovascular, and any death in eastern Finnish men." *Circulation* 91 (3):645–655, 1995.

Simon, J.A., Fong, J., Bernert, J.T., Jr., Browner, W.S. "Serum fatty acids and the risk of stroke." *Stroke* 26 (5):778–782, 1995.

Uauy-Dagach, R., Mena, P. "Nutritional role of omega-3 fatty acids during the perinatal period." *Clinical Perinatology* 22 (1):157–175, 1995.

Yang, C.Y. "Calcium and magnesium in drinking water and risk of death from cerebrovascular disease." *Stroke* 29 (2):411–414, 1998.

Temporal Lobe, Memory, and Associated Brain Damage

Barr, W.B. "Examining the right temporal lobe's role in nonverbal memory." *Brain & Cognition* 35 (1):26–41, 1997.

Becker, A., Grecksch, G. "Nootropic drugs have different effects on kindling-induced learning deficits in rats." *Pharmacological Research* 32 (3):115–122, 1995.

Blaxton, T.A., Theodore, W.H. "The role of the temporal lobes in recognizing visuospatial materials: remembering versus knowing." *Brain & Cognition* 35 (1):5–25, 1997.

Brockway, J.P., Follmer, R.L., Preuss, L.A., Prioleau, C.E., Burrows, G.S., Solsrud, K.A., Cooke, C.N., Greenhoot, J.H., Howard, J. "Memory, simple and complex language, and the temporal lobe." *Brain & Language* 61 (1):1–29, 1998.

Fleischman, D.A., Vaidya, C.J., Lange, K.L., Gabrieli, J.D. "A dissociation between perceptual explicit and implicit memory processes." *Brain & Cognition* 35 (1):42–57, 1997.

Goscinski, I., Kwiatkowski, S., Polak, J., Orlowiejska, M., Partyk, A. "The Kluver-Bucy Syndrome." *Journal of Neurosurgical Sciences* 41 (3):269–272, 1997.

Lakics, V., Sebestyen, M.G., Erdo, S.L. "Vinpocetine is a highly potent neuroprotectant against veratridine-induced cell death in primary cultures of rat cerebral cortex." *Neuroscience Letters* 185 (2):127–130, 1995.

Maguire, E.A. "Hippocampal involvement in human topographical memory: evidence from functional imaging." *Philosophical Transactions of the Royal Society of London — Series B: Biological Sciences* 352 (1360):1475–1480, 1997.

Mishkin, M., Suzuki, W.A., Gadian, D.G., Vargha-Khadem, F. "Hierarchical organization of cognitive memory. [Review]." *Philosophical Transactions of the Royal Society of London — Series B: Biological Sciences* 352 (1360):1461–1467, 1997.

Molnar, P., Erdo, S.L. "Vinpocetine is as potent as phenytoin to block voltage-gated Na+ channels in rat cortical neurons." *European Journal of Pharmacology* 273 (3):303–306, 1995.

Parker, A., Eacott, M.J., Gaffan, D. "The recognition memory deficit caused by mediodorsal thalamic lesion in un-human primates: a comparison with rhinal cortex lesion." *European Journal of Neuroscience* 9 (11):2423–2431, 1997.

Petty, R.G., Bonner, D., Mouratoglou, V., Silverman, M. "Acute frontal lobe syndrome and dyscontrol associated with bilateral caudate nucleus infarctions." *British Journal of Psychiatry* 168 (2):237–240, 1996.

Phillips, N.A., McGlone, J. "Grouped data do not tell the whole story: individual analysis of cognitive change after temporal lobectomy." *Journal of Clinical & Experimental Neuropsychology* 17 (5):713–724, 1995.

Yasuda, K., Watanabe, O., Ono, Y. "Dissociation between semantic and autobiographic memory: a case report." *Cortex* 33 (4):623–638, 1997.

Theoretical Basis for Memory Function
Cohen, T.E., Kaplan, S.W., Kandel, E.R., Hawkins, R.D. "A simplified preparation for relating cellular events to behavior: mechanisms contributing to habituation, dishabituation, and sensitization of the Aplysia gill-withdrawal reflex." *Journal of Neuroscience* 17 (8):2886–2899, 1997.

Hawkins, R.D., Cohen, T.D., Greene, W., Kandel, E.R. "Relationships between dishabituation, sensitization, and inhibition of the gill- and siphon-withdrawal reflex in Aplysia californica: effects of response measure, test time, and training stimulus." *Behavioral Neuroscience* 112 (1):24–38, 1998.

Winder, D.G., Mansuy, I.M., Osman, M., Moallem, T.M., Kandel, E.R. "Genetic and pharmacological evidence for a novel, intermediate phase of long-term potentiation suppressed by calcineurin." *Cell* 92 (1):25–37, 1998.

Transcranial Stimulation
Brandt, S.A., Ploner, C.J., Meyer, B.U. "Repetitive transcranial magnetic stimulation. Possibilities, limits and safety aspects." *Nervenarzt* 68 (10):778–784, 1997.

Chen, R., Gerloff, C., Classen, J., Wassermann, E.M., Hallett, M., Cohen, L.G. "Safety of different inter-train intervals for repetitive transcranial magnetic stimulation and recommendations for safe ranges of stimulation parameters." *Electroencephalography and Clinical Neurophysiology* 105 (6):415–421, 1997.

Haag, C., Padberg, F., Moller, H.J. "Transcranial magnetic stimulation. A diagnostic means from neurology as therapy in psychiatry?" *Nervenarzt* 68 (3):274–278, 1997.

Jahanshahi, M., Ridding, M.C., Limousin, P., Profice, P., Fogel, W., Dressler, D., Fuller, R., Brown, R.G., Brown, P., Rothwell, J.C. "Rapid rate transcranial magnetic stimulation — a safety study." *Electroencephalographic Clinical Neurophysiology* 105 (6):422–429, 1997.

Kraus, K.H., Gugino, L.D., Levy, W.J., Cadwell, J., Roth, B.J. "The use of a cap-shaped coil for transcranial magnetic stimulation of the motor cortex." *Journal of Clinical Neurophysiology* 10 (3):353–362, 1993.

Liubimskaia, I.I., Radzievskii, S.A., Bugaev, S.A., Orekhova, E.M., Gigineishvili, G.R. "The use of an electrosleep method for restoring the performance capacity and relieving the psychoemotional stress of athletes in cyclic sports." *Voprosy Kurortologii, Fizioterapii I Lechebnoi Fizicheskoi Kultury* 6:29–30, 1995.

Long, D.M. "The current status of electrical stimulation of the nervous system for the relief of chronic pain. [Review] [10 refs]." *Surgical Neurology* 49 (2):142–144, 1998.

Post, R.M., Kimbrell, T.A., McCann, U., Dunn, R.T., George, M.S., Weiss, S.R. "Are convulsions necessary for the antidepressive effect of electroconvulsive therapy: outcome of repeated transcranial magnetic stimulation." *Encephale* 23 (Spec No 3):27–35, 1997.

Wassermann, E.M., Wang, B., Zeffiro, T.A., Sadato, N., Pascual-Leone, A., Toro, C., Hallet, M. "Locating the motor cortex on the MRI with transcranial magnetic stimulation and PET." *Neuroimage* 3 (1):1–9, 1996.

Wassermann, E.M. "Risk and safety of repetitive transcranial magnetic stimulation: report and suggested guidelines from the International Workshop on the Safety of Repetitive Transcranial Magnetic Stimulation, June 5–7, 1996." *Electroencephalographic Clinical Neurophysiology* 108 (1):1–16, 1998.

Treatment for Alzheimer's Disease

Blesch, A., Tuszyanski, M. "Ex vivo gene therapy for Alzheimer's disease and spinal cord injury." *Clinical Neuroscience* 3 (5):268–274, 1995–96.

Drachman, D.A., Leber, P. "Treatment of Alzheimer's disease — searching for a breakthrough, settling for less." *New England Journal of Medicine* 336 (17):1241–1247, 1997.

Evans, D.A., Morris, M.C. "Is a randomized trial of antioxidants in the primary prevention of Alzheimer's disease warranted?" *Alzheimer's Disease & Associated Disorders* 10 (Suppl 1):45–49, 1996.

Farlow, M.R., Lahiri, D.K., Poirer, J., Davignon, J., Schneider, L., Hui, S.L. "Treatment outcome of tacrine therapy depends on apolipoprotein genotype and gender of the subjects with Alzheimer's disease." *Neurology* 50 (3):669–677, 1998.

Freedman, M., Rewilak, D., Xerri, T., Cohen, S., Gordon, A.S., Shandling, M., Logan, A.G. "L-deprenyl in Alzheimer's disease: cognitive and behavioral effects." *Neurology* 50 (3):660–668, 1998.

Glasky, A.J., Glasky, M.S., Ritzman, R.F., Rathbone, M.P. "AIT-082, a novel purine derivative with neuro regenerative properties." *Experimental Opinion Investigative Drugs* 6 (10):1413–1417, 1997.

Gray, S. "Advertisements for donepezil (Aricept) in the BMJ: Advertisement suggests an unrealistic improvement in mental status." *British Medical Journal* 314 (7093):1555, 1997.

Henderson, V.W. "The epidemiology of estrogen replacement therapy and Alzheimer's disease." *Neurology* 48 (5, Suppl 7): S27–35, 1997.

Lawlor, B.A., Aisen, P.S., Green, C., Fine, E., Schmeidler, J. "Selegiline in the treatment of behavioural disturbance in Alzheimer's disease." *International Journal of Geriatric Psychiatry* 12 (3):319–322, 1997.

Lendavai, B., Sershen, H., Lajtha, A., Santha, E., Barany, M., Vizi, E.S. "Differential mechanisms involved in the effect of nicotinic agonists DMPP and lobeline to release [3H] 5-HT from rat hippocampal slices." *Neuropharmacology* 35 (12):1769–1777, 1996.

Lewin, E.D., Rose, J.E., Abood, L. "Effects of nicotinic dimethylaminoethyl esters on working memory performance of rats in the radial-arm maze." *Pharmacology, Biochemistry and Behavior* 51 (2–3):369–373, 1995.

Mackenzie, I.R., Munoz, D.G. "Nonsteroidal anti-inflammatory drug use and Alzheimer-type pathology in aging." *Neurology* 50 (4):986–990, 1998.

Rao, T.S., Correa, L.D., Lloyd, G.K. "Effects of lobeline and dimethylphenylpiperazinium iodide (DMPP) on N-methyl-D-asparatate (NMDA)-evoked acetylcholine release in vitro: evidence from lack of involvement of classical neuronal nicotinic acetylcholine receptors." *Neuropharmacology* 36 (1):39–50, 1997.

Raskind, M.A., Sadowsky, C.H., Sigmund, W.R., Beitler, P.J., Auster, S.B. "Effect of tacrine on language, praxis and noncognitive behavioral problems in Alzheimer's disease." *Archives of Neurology* 54 (7):836–840, 1997.

Rathbone, M.P., Middlemiss, P., Craig, A., Caciagliagli, F., Ciccarelli, R., DiIozo, P., Huang, R. "The trophic effects of Purines and purinergic signaling in pathologic reactions of astrocytes." *Alzheimer Disease and Associated Disorders* 3, Suppl 2:536–545, 1998.

Rogers, S.L., Friedhoff, L.T. "The efficacy and safety of donepezil in patients with Alzheimer's disease: results of a US Multicentre, Randomized, Double-Blind, Placebo-Controlled Trial. The Donepezil Study Group." *Dementia* 7 (6):293–303, 1996.

Rogers, S.L., Farlow, M.R., Doody, R.S., Mohs, R., Friedhoff, L.T. "A 24-week, double-blind, placebo-controlled trial of donepezil in patients with Alzheimer's disease. Donepezil Study Group." *Neurology* 50 (1):136–145, 1998.

Sano, M., Ernesto, C., Thomas, R.G., Klauber, M.R., Schafer, K., Grundman, M., Woodbury, P., Growdon, J., Cotman, C.W., Pfeiffer, E., Schneider, L.S., Thal, L.J. "A controlled trial of selegiline, alpha-tocopherol, or both as treatment for Alzheimer's disease. The Alzheimer's Disease Cooperative Society." *New England Journal of Medicine* 336 (17):1216–1222, 1997.

Schneider, L.S., Farlow, M. "Combined tacrine and estrogen replacement therapy in patients with Alzheimer's disease." *Annals of the New York Academy of Sciences* 826:317–322, 1997.

Small, G.W., Rabins, P.V., Barry, P.P., Buckholts, N.S., DeKosky, S.T., Ferris, S.H., Finkel, S.I., Gwyther, L.P., Khachaturian, Z.S., Lebowitz, B.D., McRae, T.D., Morris, J.C., Oakley, F., Schneider, L.S., Streim, J.E., Suderland, T., Teri, L.A., Tune, L.E. "Diagnosis and treatment of Alzheimer's disease and related disorders. Consensus Statement of the American Association for Geriatric Psychiatry, the Alzheimer's Association, and the American Geriatrics Society." *Journal of American Medical Association* 278 (16):1363–1371, 1997.

Steward, W.F., Jawas, C., Corrada, M., Metter, E.J. "Risk of Alzheimer's disease and duration of NSAID use." *Neurology* 48 (3):626–632, 1997.

Zemlan, F.P. "Velnacrine for the treatment of Alzheimer's disease: a double-blind, placebo-controlled trial. The Mentane Study Group." *Journal of Neural Transmission* 103 (8–9):1105–1116, 1996.

Index

Acetylcholine, 258, 268; in memory process, 101, 132, 141, 146, 255–56, 287. *See also* Neurotransmitters

Acid-base balance, 163–64, 168

Acronym-building, 29

Actovegin (blood derivative), 284

Adams, Ray, 150

Age, 3, 4, 39–40, 68–86; and brain disorders, 203, 204, 208, (Alzheimer's) 247, 250, 259, 263–64, (hydrocephalus) 241–43, (subdural hematoma), 236–37; and CAT scans, 222; and depression (severe), 97–101, 186; and DHEAS, 186; and diet supplements (vitamins), 148, 157, 228; and electrolyte balance, 158, 161, 162, 167; and epileptic seizures, 211; kinds of memory affected by, 70; and medication, 100, (dosage) 128, 133, 142; and memory loss, 3, 4, 39–40, 68–86, 293, (national policy) 81–83; and misdiagnosis, 182; and new vs. old learning, 69; and pernicious anemia, 157; recovery time for, 133; research studies on, 68–71; and stroke prevention, 232

AIDS (autoimmune deficiency syndrome), 196, 197, 200, 201; and memory loss, 198–99

Air bags, need for, 208, 267, 285

Alcohol: as brain poison, 61, 111–21, 148–51, 267, (and Alzheimer's) 248, 266, (and strokes) 219, 226, 231; combined with other drugs, 120; and depression, 91–92, 105; and memory loss, 23, 66, 113–16, 127, 149–51, (reversible) 78; and misdiagnosis of alcoholism, 182, 187; myths concerning, 116–20; red wine, 119, 231–32, 284; seizures caused by, 78, 114, 117, 209; vital points to remember, 121; and vitamin B-1 deficiency, 23, 43, 78, 114, 116, 148–51

Alcoholics Anonymous, 121, 130

Alcohol industry, 148–49, 151

Alexander the Great, 117

Alpha-tocopherol. *See* Vitamin E

Aluminum as risk factor, 248, 265–66

Alzheimer's disease, 246–60; age and, 247, 259, 263–64, (age of onset) 250; aluminum and, 248, 265–66; brain injury and, 266; causes of, 247–48, (beta amyloid protein theory) 247, 249, 286, 287; choline and, 146, 248, 255–56; and competence/incompetence, 77–78, 86, 255, 259; depression mistaken for, 75–77, 97–98; difficulty in diagnosing, 70–71, 196, 249, 250–51, 259; diseases associated with, 264–65, (hydrocephalus) 243; genetics and, 247, 248, 259, 263; hypothyroidism mistaken for, 182–83, 184, 187; international conference on (1998), 257; myths about, 247; prevention of, 284; and reversal of memory loss, 190, 253, 258–59, (nicotine and) 282–83, (predicted) 286–88; reversible complications of, 251, 259; risk factors, 71, 248, 265–69; seizures mistaken for, 211, 212;

Index

Brain injuries (cont.)
ory loss, 18, 30, 189–90; open-head injuries, 203; prevention of, 266–69, 285; post-mortem examination of, 23; and reversal of memory loss, *See* Memory loss reversal; surgery for, 235–45; tumors, 42–43, 81, 114, 213, 238–41, 245; vital points to remember, 201, 208, 244–45. *See also* Epileptic seizures; Strokes
Brain Power (Mark and Mark), 178, 279
Bush, George H. W., 139n
Butters, Nelson, 116
B vitamins. *See* Vitamin B group

California health studies, 186, 275–76
Cambridge (England) vitamin study, 229
Cantab (computerized test), 47
Carbon monoxide poisoning, 107
Case Western Reserve University Alzheimer's center, 282–83
CAT (computerized axial tomography) scan: diagnosing brain disorders, 115, 199, 213, 236, 237–38, 240–45 *passim*; diagnosing strokes, 218, 219, 222, 226, 227; how it works, 34; need for, 85, 195; testing memory, 81
Center for Memory Impairment and Neurobehavioral Disturbances (CMIND), 80–81, 140
Centers for Disease Control and Prevention, 230–31
Cerebellum, 13, 14, 15 (fig.)
Cerebral infarctions, 23
Cerebrovascular and cardiovascular disease: studies of, 229–30, 231. *See also* Brain injuries/disorders
Cerebrum, 13 (fig.), 15, 17 (fig.)
Chiles, Allan, 290
Choline, 146, 248, 255–56; as diet supplement, 146, 270n, 271–73
Cholinergic neurotransmitters, 101n, 255. *See also* Acetylcholine
Cholinesterases (enzymes), 256
"Chunking" of information, 22
Churchill, Winston, 117
Cigarettes. *See* Tobacco
Cimetidine (prescription drug), 139, 268
Cingulum, 15, 16 (fig.)
Circadian rhythms, 181. *See also* Sleep
Citocoline, 272–73. *See also* Choline
Cocaine. *See* Street drugs
Coffee, 122, 126–27, 130

Cognitive Diagnostics, Inc., 46–47
"Cognometer," 46, 47
Compazine (tranquilizer), 135
Competence/incompetence, Alzheimer's disease and, 77–78, 86, 255, 259
Concentration: lack of (hyperdistractibility), 65, 93, 105, 187, 290, 292; in memory process, 27–28, 29–30, 32
Conditioned reflexes, 10, 55, 67; athletes' loss of, 34, 60–61; bad, and memory loss, 51–53, 54, 56, 61, 63–66; and cortisol levels, 64; music and, 62–63; Pavlovian, 51, 186; and relaxation programs, 280; and sleep, 108
Confabulation, 150
Coronary disease: alcohol or diet and, 119, 231, 232–34; strokes related to, 232–33
Cortisol levels, 64, 65, 185–86
Cyclotron, definition of, 35

Danish sleep study, 108
Dehydration. *See* Water
Dementia: alcohol-related, 266; causes of, 191, 192; degenerative (with Lewy bodies), 252; diagnosis and treatment of, 68, 70, 79, 197, 259; misdiagnosis of, 89, 200, 211, 252; multi-infarct, 215–21, 234, 288; treatable, with Alzheimer's, 259
Deprenyl (inhibitor drug), 256–57
Depression: brain chemistry and, 90, 100, 105; brain injury and, 205; classifications of, 89–90; clinical, 90–92; and cognitive reaction time, 46; cortisol levels and, 64, 65; manic-depressive illness, 125; medication for, *See* Medication, prescription; and memory loss, 87–105, 290, 292, (reversibility of) 88, 101, 105, 186, 250; misdiagnosis of, 182, 200, 240; mistaken for Alzheimer's or dementia, 75–77, 89, 97–98; severe, 95–97, (in the elderly) 97–101, 186; street drugs and, 91–92, 123; stress-induced, 89–90, 101–5; stroke-related, 226, 227; studies of, 186–87; and suicide, 95–97, 99n; testing for, 80–81, 85, (memory test patterns) 44, 45; therapy for, 92, 96–97, 105, 186, (electrical brain stimulation) 101, 289–90 (*See also* medication for, above; vital memory points to remember, 105; worsens memory problem, 38, 51, 78, 88–89, 90, 93–95, 219
Desyrel (antidepressant), 222

334

Index

Index

Index